FEED YOUR BODY
RIGHT

—— **From Birth to Adulthood** ——

ALBERT C. GOLDBERG, MD, MS, FAAP

FEED YOUR BODY
RIGHT

— From Birth to Adulthood —

CFI

An imprint of Cedar Fort, Inc.
Springville, Utah

ISBN 13: 978-1-4621-3939-2

Published by CFI, an imprint of Cedar Fort, Inc.
2373 W. 700 S., Springville, UT 84663
Distributed by Cedar Fort, Inc., www.cedarfort.com

Library of Congress Control Number: 2020948521

Cover design by Courtney Proby
Cover design © 2021 Cedar Fort, Inc.
Edited by Valene Wood

Printed in the United States of America

10 9 8 7 6 5 4 3 2 1

Printed on acid-free paper

Dedication

I am often asked, "Why did you become a pediatrician?" To answer this question: I dedicate this book to my son Keith Goldberg, who was poisoned within the safety of his mother's womb by a drug called Thalidomide.[1]

December 11, 1961–June 14, 1962

Contents

CONTENTS

Introduction

How the Food Industry Purposely Fogs
Your Understanding of Nutrition

At the beginning of the 20th century, malnutrition—the lack of certain nutrients, vitamins, and minerals—was a problem second only to infection
in this country. Today, malnutrition is more likely to be a case of overconsumption of certain nutrients. Too much has replaced too little—too much
fat, too much salt, too much sugar, and too much ultra-processed food. In
this book I will reveal the solutions to the problems of overconsumption.
The book is peppered throughout with helpful examples of what foods
to avoid (but not totally eliminate) and with notes on what to look out for
when reading the packages of your favorite foods.

My suggestions and anecdotes come from years of experience as a
pediatrician in Marin County, California, nurturing thousands of children
(and their parents), and from the experience of many other experts in
nutrition. For the past 35 years I have worked in almost all countries in
South and Central America, India, China, Nepal, Bangladesh, Vietnam,
Philippines, Myanmar (Burma), Egypt, and Ethiopia. These are countries
where poverty, ignorance, social disintegration, and war have contributed
to nutritional disease. From there I brought back a keen understanding
of the multicultural effects of diet or the food choices made by parents,
children, adolescents, and adults.

In Central and South America I've seen and treated all the classic
nutritional diseases including rickets, scurvy, pellagra, and kwahiorkor.[2]
I've witnessed the nutritional changes taking place in China, the Philippines, and India with its high white rice diet now associated with a surge
in type 2 diabetes, and where the introduction of the Western diet has
made heart disease a new leading cause of death in their countries
replacing infectious disease.[3]

I have learned from practical experience that it is not easy to alter
a person's food choices. Change involves much more than presenting

nation or making healthier food available. There are many
involved in food choice or selection, such as one's reli-
ground, ethnicity, one's inherited temperament, and of
ty of competing low-priced sugary and salty snacks.
er of five plus twelve grandchildren and a pediatrician in
practice for over thirty-five years, I've been in a good position to
witness how the average American family's diet stacks up. There has
been a major shift in our children's dietary habits. Fewer families eat their
dinner meal together. I have found that eating meals together as a family
has increased our children's consumption of fruits and vegetables. The
health advantages to children who eat with a family add more lasting
value above and beyond nutrition.

Nutrition has been an area of great interest to me since before medical school. As a student at Muhlenberg College, in Allentown, Pennsylva-
nia, I visited Rodale's farm[4] and learned about his organic farming while
taking one of the country's first college-level courses on Conservation.
Rachel Carson's *Silent Spring* had just been published and it gave me
further insight into the long-term effects of what we eat and environmental consequences of DDT. After reading Nathan Pritikin's *Live Longer
Now* and Campbell's *China Study,* I realized how much more I needed
to learn about dietary theories that conflict with the traditional nutritional
curriculum. Nutrition, as taught in medical school, was a small part of the
our biochemistry and physiology curriculum. While extremely important,
there was little practical nutrition. I learned what was scientifically known
at the time about digestion of foods, carbohydrates, fats, proteins, minerals, and vitamins. These classes gave me a fundamental understanding
of how our body works and the tools to understand the merits of a good
diet as well as the pitfalls of fad diets. I will pass this information on to
you in my important chapter called "The Chemicals of Life: Nutrition 101."

Most physicians share the concerns over the pesticides used in
growing fruit and vegetables plus the new and old additives incorporated
into our convenience foods. These issues are discussed in the chapter
"Food Additives and Environmental Contaminants." This will describe in
depth the most worrisome food contaminants—residual chemicals used
by farmers to increase production of fish, crustaceans, shell foods, as
well as endocrine modulators.

In 2019 Marin County was ranked the healthiest county in California
for the ninth time in ten years by an annual survey conducted by the
University of Wisconsin Population Health Institute and the Robert Wood
Johnson Foundation.[5] It evaluates counties across the nation to measure

how healthy residents are and how long they live. However, if you follow the county by zip codes, you will find that the healthiest sectors are where the wealthiest and most educated families live. Those families smoked less, exercised more regularly, and consumed a diet higher in fresh fruit and vegetables. The zip codes that represented the poorest neighborhoods, scored the worst, and represented families with the lowest incomes and less educational achievement. There are fewer grocery stores with fresh fruit and vegetables available in their part of town. Obesity is rampant and parents are often afraid to send their children outside to play because of fear from the ICE (U.S. Immigration and Customs Enforcement) and few safe play areas.

The Covid-19 pandemic has magnified these distortions and inequities for those who were most negatively affected: children who are overweight or obese and adults with the consequences of a lifetime of poor eating choices—diabetes, hypertension, strokes, and cardiovascular diseases. These events need not be an inherent part of the "aging" process.

This book contains everything a parent or adult needs to know in order to design an optimal diet for the well child—from infancy through the teenage years and adulthood. When you find out about sodium, for instance, no matter what your age or family medical history, I believe you'll be grateful for my Five-Step Program to cut down the amount of salt or sodium in your diet. It is important to make changes in manageable steps, and come up with foods that are acceptable in your household.

Feed Your Body Right from Birth through Adulthood will help you find your way through the thicket of nutritional information, the hype and the misinformation that's out there. It will surely have an effect on your eating habits and will improve the health of children and adult readers.

There is a special need for a practical and honest nutrition book that contains evidence-based information rather than faith-based thinking passed off as "science." Much of the nutritional information handed down to us is not evidence based, without bias or a hidden agenda. It is what we were taught by our parents, grandparents, and professors at medical school. This is what I mean by "faith-based." In addition, there are many dietary laws drawn from religions that are blindly followed by orthodox members. No problem there, but it is vital that you are aware of the non-scientific source of your information.

Feed Your Body Right from Birth through Adulthood addresses the daily nutritional health issues of children and adults in a specific, scientific, and friendly way. It is not a "diet book," such as a "weight loss" book. This is my attempt to help you prevent the onset of child obesity, early cardiovascular disease, metabolic syndrome, diabetes, and those illnesses falsely referred to as diseases of aging.

I hope you will find yourself returning to this book over and over again. It will help you sort through exaggerations and distortions manufactured by the mainstream food industry and "health food" industry specifically designed to confuse you, and make you distrust all nutritional information.

Chapters will be devoted to the practical issues such as breastfeeding, picky eaters, eating out, fast food restaurants, and ideas for school lunches.

In addition to parents, this book will be of special interest to nursery schools, elementary and high school teachers, coaches, all healthcare providers, family physicians, pediatricians, and nurse practitioners.

CHAPTER 1

The Food Industry Fogs Your Understanding of Nutrition

One of the most important duties of physicians and healthcare practitioners is to teach families what they can do to prevent future health-related illness. I fully recognize that it is a tall order and extremely time-consuming for medical practitioners who work for profit-driven medical offices and corporations. But, remember, "Doctor" means teacher, and it's their obligation to teach patients that food is the most potent first medicine.

Most doctors' offices are repair shops, trying to correct the damage caused by poor lifestyles, poor nutrition, and social inequity. It is my hope that more doctors join with others to improve the delivery of medical care in the USA and defog the distortions, half truths, and outright lies promoted by the Food Industry.

In 1967, as medical director and nutritional advisor of the first Head Start Program in Marin County, California, I developed its initial medical and nutrition program. This experience taught me how diet can improve minds as well as bodies. It is unfortunate that the well-intentioned school lunch programs subsidized by the US Department of Agriculture were turned into a dumping ground for fat, high sodium, high-sugar juices, and low-fiber foods. Under the Reagan administration, ketchup was actually legislated to be a vegetable choice.[6] The fresh fruit supplied by schools was so under-ripe and tasteless that sadly most children just ended up tossing it in the garbage. More recently, many improvements have been made after concerned parents organized and pressured their local and congressional representatives.

An entire industry has matured in the past few years, scamming the gullible and naive public by promoting and selling several types of water. I will discuss a few below, but first a brief discussion on water.

WATER

Keeping well-hydrated is crucial for health and well-being. There is no universally agreed upon quantity of water that must be consumed daily. Most people rely on thirst as a mechanism for how much water to consume, but this is not a reliable method. Older adults gradually lose their sense of thirstiness and can easily become dehydrated without realizing it. Infants and children can quickly become dehydrated with vomiting and diarrhea. Water is essential for the kidneys and other bodily functions.

Severe cases of dehydration can lead to kidney and heart failure.

Water lubricates the joints and forms saliva and mucus as well as regulating body temperature. The digestive system needs water as it makes minerals and nutrients accessible besides boosting performance during exercise.

These are but a few of the needs for water. After all, adults are 60% and our blood is 90% water.

In addition to drinking fluids, about 20–30% comes from the food we eat, such as soups, milk, fruit, and vegetables.

Drinking tested water from the tap is the safest and least expensive source of fluid for the body.

Plastic disposable water bottles are so popular that the empty bottles have become a major cause of river and ocean pollution. Be kind to Mother Earth and use a reusable water bottle.

RAW WATER

Raw water is unfiltered, unprocessed, or untreated water that is bottled directly from a natural spring. Some companies are selling this water and marketing it as a safer alternative to chemically-treated water. Their position is that this water has natural probiotics that help promote digestion and good health. Raw water does not offer distinct health benefits over drinking tap water. Supporters of raw water believe that sterilizing and purifying water destroys the natural minerals and probiotics present in water. Before the development of public water systems and water treatment centers, waterborne illnesses, such as typhoid and cholera, were not uncommon. Now how can I keep an "open mind" on this one? *Caveat Emptor.* You be the judge.

PROTEIN WATER

Protein water, which has an added whey protein isolate, is promoted as a low calorie protein drink and a superior hydration beverage. A supporting study was made and funded by the Protein Water Industry.

DEEP OCEAN WATER

Deep ocean water is desalinated water from a deep ocean current. The brand "Kona Deep Water" claims that this water has a unique blend of electrolytes and trace minerals that hydrates you twice as fast as bottled spring water. There's nothing special about Kona Deep, except the price. It is basically just water.

HYDROGEN WATER

Hydrogen water is water with added molecules of hydrogen. The promotors claim it "Boosts endurance, minimizes lactic acid, and reduces fatigue" and promises to improve athletic performance, reduce inflammation, and deliver powerful antioxidants. There is no evidence to back up the claims for hydrogen water.[7]

"IONIZED" AND "ALKALINE" WATER

I have strong feelings about this, so I won't go into detail about it. For those interested in this matter, I refer you to the websites: www.chem1.com/CQ/ionbunk.html and www.quackwatch.org.[8]

ICE WATER

One more word about drinking water, that is, ice water with a meal. You may have been advised not to drink ice water with a meal. The explanation is that it damages your body's ability to properly digest food and drink. Food goes down improperly digested and the body is unable to retrieve the nutrients and energy that it needs. They claim that by decreasing the activity of your digestive system, cold beverages rob you of the nutrition of the food and that your body has to use energy in order to warm up that liquid inside your body. These pseudo-nutritionists proclaim further, without a shred of evidence, that the immune system, which works to fight off colds and other illnesses, can also suffer from this incomplete digestion because it does not have the energy it needs to function correctly. It is important to look for science-based evidence for hypotheses like this one. Far too many are fooled by these illogical ideas. This cold water advice was introduced to me in earnest by a Board Certified Plastic Surgeon. Go figure!

Bottom Line: Don't waste your time or money on these water gimmicks.

SALT: IS IT TRULY THE WHITE DEATH?

Salt, or sodium chloride, is one of our oldest food preservatives, used in commercially prepared foods as an inexpensive way to inhibit molds, retard spoilage, and provide smooth texture and quick-cooking properties. It's also a necessary mineral in our diet. On food labels, the words sodium, soda, monosodium glutamate, or the chemical symbol for sodium, Na, all signify salt. An infant's preference for salt does not emerge until four months, but how much is innate and how much is learned remains uncertain—quite unlike our taste for sugar, with which we seem to be inborn.[9]

Too much salt in childhood is an extreme dietary hazard, and has been linked to the development of hypertension (high blood pressure) in teenagers and adults. A high-salt diet beginning in infancy is a major cause of high blood pressure in adulthood. In a Dutch study, newborns who were fed, in addition to breast milk, formula and foods providing 22mg of sodium a day had lower blood pressures than those fed diets with 58 mg a day. Fifteen years after the study ended, the difference in blood pressure was still there.[10]

While high blood pressure seems to run in some families genetically, lots of sodium helps encourage this undesirable family trait. Whether or not there is any history of high blood pressure or stroke in your family, I recommend you limit your child's sodium intake—and your own.

The amount of sodium in a diet should approximate a ratio of sodium in milligrams (mg) to the amount of calories in your diet. In other words, a 700-calorie diet should have sodium limited to about 700mg while a 2000-calorie diet should limit sodium intake to 2000mg or two grams. Avoid foods with more than 350 mg of sodium per serving. The right amount of sodium needed by children through adulthood can be found *naturally* in fresh vegetables, grains, meats, poultry, and fish. But in fact, many children consume over 5000 mg of sodium daily. Adults often consume from 10,000 to 12,000 milligrams *daily* between what's natural in the food, what the food industry has added to the food, and what we add ourselves from the salt shaker in the kitchen and at the table!

Speaking of the Food industry, there have been a few studies, mostly subsidized by the Food Industry, claiming that the effect of sodium as a cause of high blood pressure has been greatly exaggerated. The researchers are from reputable universities, but these seriously flawed studies have been very short term. Totally ignored in these studies are infants, children, and young adults. Newspapers, magazines, and "health journals" have been complicit in publishing outrageous distortions under headlines suggesting salt should be used more liberally and that our prior understanding of salt or sodium is now, can you believe this, "obsolete dogma." No wonder most people are confused when presented with such misinformation. Chefs from major restaurants are already featuring dishes "enhanced with flavors from exotic healthy salts."

I have actually heard many pediatricians say, "Don't worry about salt or sodium, it is an important part of the diet." Then they cite only rare salt-losing diseases such as Addison's disease, cystic fibrosis, or another rare problem found in some children and teenagers who suffer from fainting due to low blood pressure. This nutritional perversion does not negate the truth of salt producing hypertension. This is what the Food Industry is promoting so effectively.[11]

High blood pressure is a serious matter. What a child eats sets the stage for high blood pressure later in life. It can eventually lead to heart failure, a condition where the heart gets larger and weaker and is less able to pump blood. High blood pressure (hypertension) can also lead to aneurisms. Aneurisms are small blister-like areas in the blood vessels of the brain (leading to a stroke) or the aorta, which can burst (dissecting aortic artery), causing sudden rapid death or permanent disability. Kidney failure is another result of high blood pressure. As blood vessels in the kidney narrow, they are less able to supply the kidney w'   ᵈ This could lead to permanent kidney damage. Hypertension aᶥ the hardening of arteries. Healthy arteries are elastic. When⁄ to the brain, heart, and other organs in the body become ⏀ hard, they are less able to carry blood and the result is⁄ premature death of these organs.

A stroke is a "brain attack" and its mechanism is similar to a "heart attack." Blood to the brain either becomes blocked (the most common type) and is referred to as an "ischemic stroke," or bursts and is referred to as a "hemorrhagic stroke." In both cases, damage to the brain is caused by lack of oxygen and blood glucose. Oxygen and glucose (sugar) are essential nutrients carried to the brain by blood vessels. Brain cells quickly begin to die without these nutrients. The results may be impaired speech if the brain cells in the speech center die; paralysis of the arms or legs if the motor brain cells die; blindness if the vision center brain cells die; or coma and death if the stroke is severe enough to cause the death of enough vital brain cells. A diet low in sodium, saturated fat, and added sugar, plus regular exercise greatly reduces the risk of stroke. Although stroke is usually an event that occurs in adulthood, its roots (poor food choices and exercise habits) are developed during childhood.

When selecting a food, note the amount of calories. Then check the label for sodium content. If the sodium content in milligrams is far above the number of calories, search the shelves for a brand that contains less salt. There are many canned soups available now that have a reduced or low salt counterpart. Bread and cheese are very high salt foods. Check the labels—you'll be surprised. Take time out one day to calculate how much salt you actually consume in a day. The figure may be shocking!

For most Americans, 10% of the sodium in their diet occurs naturally in food, 15% comes from the salt they shake on while cooking or at the table, and 75% is added to food during processing. A bowl of canned chicken noodle soup can deliver 900 mg of sodium—for a child, that's over a day's worth of sodium and that's why it's so important to check the Nutrition Facts label.

Children in a nationally representative sample consumed an average of 3,387 mgs of sodium per day, more than double the upper limit of 1500 mgs recommended.

The Recommended Dietary Allowance (RDA) of sodium for healthy adults is 2,300 mg daily. That is equivalent to one teaspoon (6375mg) of salt a day. The children's RDA for sodium are the following:

Ages 2–3 are 1000 mgs
Ages 4–8 are 1200 mgs
Ages 9–18 are 1500 mgs

If you can save your child from the habit of craving a relatively high diet, you may save him or her from future heart disease or stroke, or an earlier death. I personally know many middle-aged men and women who ignored this advice and have suffered possibly preventable brain-damaging strokes.

A cup of cottage cheese, a small bag of pretzels, and a salad with Italian dressing contains more than the adult recommended daily limit of sodium—2400 mg! A glass serving of Campbell's 100% tomato juice contains 980 mg of sodium and the parmesan cheese sprinkled on top of the pasta dinner adds about 500 mg.

Improve your odds by modifying your own salt intake. The following is a five-step program for the gradual reduction of salt in your family's diet. It takes most adults about a year to withdraw from the salt craving. Go slowly and you won't feel deprived. It will take the children much less time, but in either case it's a minor and brief deprivation in the big scheme of things, and worth it.

FIVE STEPS FOR MODIFYING SALT INTAKE

1. Empty the salt from the shaker on the table and refill with a non-sodium herbal substitute.

2. Gradually use less salt in cooking—don't use it at all in cooking water. Start with half the salt a recipe calls for. After a few months, omit salt from cooking entirely.

3. Notice sodium content on food labels. Decrease your sodium intake to below 2,300 milligrams if you are an adult, or less if you are younger (refer to the RDA above). Remember: if you consume 2,000 calories a day, your sodium intake should equal 2,000mg or less per day. This is an easy "rule of thumb" to remember. Calories per day=Milligrams of sodium per day. Canned foods are very high in sodium (unless specifically stated as, "reduced sodium, low sodium or no salt added"), followed by frozen foods, but some fresh foods are too—like tomato and celery—therefore don't add salt to such dishes. Stop buying canned soups! These are "hypertension in a can." Eat fresh fruit daily to supply much needed potassium to balance your sodium intake.

4. Don't keep highly salted foods in the house. Avoid the temptation of buying high sodium crackers, chips, salted nuts, bacon, sausages, lunch meats, dehydrated soups, tomato or V-8 juice, most canned soups, pickles, relishes, barbecue sauces, lox, herring, many processed cheeses

and especially cheddar cheeses, or Jell-O. Treat yourself to such foods only on special occasions in small amounts, when you're away from home or at a Super Bowl party.

5.   In a year's time you won't believe how different foods taste or that you ever purposefully put salt on your corn on the cob! Restaurant food may seem very salty, unless you ask the chef to use very little salt and no MSG.

There are other measures that help control hypertension. Exercise regularly; make this a daily routine and keep it a part of your lifestyle as you do with brushing your teeth. Lose weight and keep it off by eating smaller portions. You may need to take medication for the rest of your life to keep your blood pressure in a safe range. Do not despair! The earlier you begin these lifestyle changes, the better chance those future "Golden Years" will have to become truly Golden.

THE PROCESSED (SALT) FOOD INDUSTRY SPEAKS UP[12]

By Fiona Godlee
Author affiliations
Assistant editor, BMJ London WC1H 9JR
(British Medical Journal)
Delaying salt reductions has public health and commercial costs

"Like any group with vested interests, the food industry resists regulation. Faced with a growing scientific consensus that salt increases blood pressure and the fact that most dietary salt (65–85%) comes from processed foods, some of the world's major food manufacturers have adopted desperate measures to try to stop governments from recommending salt reduction. Rather than reformulate their products, manufacturers have lobbied governments, refused to cooperate with expert working parties, encouraged misinformation campaigns, and tried to discredit the evidence. This week's BMJ finds them defending their interests as vigorously as ever.

"In 1988 the BMJ published data from the Intersalt study suggesting that populations with high average intakes of salt were likely to have higher average systolic blood pressures and that salt intake predicted rise in blood pressure with age. The salt producers' international trade organization, the Salt Institute, criticized the study, particularly the methods used to relate blood pressure to age, and asked the investigators to hand over their raw data for reanalysis. The investigators instead performed the reanalyses themselves: these confirmed the previous findings."

WHAT'S ALL THIS TALK ABOUT SUGAR?

THE SUGAR HYPOTHESIS

Sugar as a cause of cardiovascular disease, was reported by Dr. Hohn Yudkin in Lancet, a respected British Medical Journal, in 1964. Yudkin studied levels of dietary sucrose (table sugar) in patients with coronary atherosclerotic (hardening of the blood vessels) disease. He claimed that dietary sugar might be involved causally in coronary heart disease and type 2 diabetes. In another study that followed, it was shown that the sugar intake of men with heart attacks or artery disease was twice that of others without cardiovascular disease. Studies he conducted on sugar indicated that they raised blood triglycerides and insulin levels. Dr. Yudkin's claims were pushed aside when subsequent studies did not confirm the original claims that sucrose was a major contributor to coronary heart disease risk.

Investigators and endocrinologists are still claiming simple sugars, especially sucrose, fructose, and high fructose corn syrup (HFCS) to be the culprits involved in our epidemic of obesity, diabetes type 2, and cardiovascular disease (The Metabolic Syndrome). In 1972 Dr. Yudkin's book *Pure, White, and Deadly* was published by Davis-Poynter Ltd. *Sweet and Dangerous* was published in 1972 by Bantam Books. Read what happened and how this study was debunked.

HAVE THEY NO SHAME?

Anahad O'Connor of the New York Times wrote, "The sugar industry paid scientists in the 1960s to play down the link between sugar and heart disease and promote saturated fat as the culprit instead, newly released historical documents show."[13]

The internal sugar industry documents, recently discovered by a researcher at the University of California, San Francisco, and published in JAMA Internal Medicine, suggest that five decades of research into the role of nutrition and heart disease, including many of today's dietary recommendations, may have been largely shaped by the sugar industry.

"They were able to derail the discussion about sugar for decades," said Stanton Glantz, a professor of medicine at U.C.S.F. and an author of the JAMA Internal Medicine paper.

The documents show that a trade group called the Sugar Research Foundation, known today as the Sugar Association, paid three Harvard scientists the equivalent of about $50,000 in today's dollars to publish a 1967 review of research on sugar, fat, and heart disease. The studies used in the review were handpicked by the sugar group, and the article, which was published in the prestigious New England Journal of Medicine, minimized the link between sugar and heart health and cast aspersions on the role of saturated fat.[14]

THE "HEALTH FOOD INDUSTRY," THE 21ST CENTURY SNAKE OIL

There are few short cuts to good nutrition. Each week a new herbal, vitamin or mineral is featured at the health food store promising the consumer greater longevity and a clearer, more facile mind. This approach is specifically derived from soft evidence suggesting some benefits from an amino acid, vitamin, mineral, or herb and sold as a panacea. These products are very iffy at best. As an example, beta carotene taken as a supplement by smokers actually increased morbidity and mortality due to lung cancer instead of giving the assumed protection.[15] I am not saying that supplements are not important. They definitely are. Particularly Vitamin D, folic acid, Vitamin B-12 (especially in the elderly and vegan/vegetarians), B-6 in certain select groups, calcium, and selenium. But there is little evidence that these nutrients help very much if the consumer consumes a balanced diet high in fiber, low in sodium and saturated fats.

To get the protective effect of these nutrients, you must eat adequate amounts of fruits and vegetables every day. Foods work together in concert. Isolating any of the many nutritional compounds and putting them in pill form unfortunately causes them to lose most of their effectiveness for reasons that are not totally clear. Save your money and buy the real thing! All those "nutrients" and antioxidants won't make up for a fatty, salty, sugary diet that is low in fruits and vegetables.

SUPPLEMENTS AND "MEDICAL FOODS"

The Health Food Industry is always interested in increasing profits. This multibillion-dollar industry's answer is supplements and more recently, "medical foods."[16] vitamins and minerals in the form of pills, capsules, and powders are promoted to "make sure" nutrition is complete. The mantra is, "just to be sure" that your poor diet or picky eater's diet is nutritionally complete. "Health Food" stores promote all types of antioxidants to their clients in beverage or pill form as nutritional supplements, overstating their power to prevent heart attacks, correct erectile dysfunction (ED), support the immune system, fight inflammation, and unlock health secrets of "Traditional Chinese Herbal Medicine." Many of these clients thus continue their lethal dietary habit of consuming a high saturated fat, high simple sugar, highly refined food, fried food, and high salt diet. Each year the "Health Food Industry" comes up with a new "Fountain of Youth."

"Supports" is the magical word that permits those claims to be legal. By using this phrase "helps support," as long as the claims do not name a disease or promise to treat a condition, they are able to get around regulations, and hype their pills based on pseudoscience. This multi-billion dollar industry is the 21st century Snake Oil.

The Food and Drug Administration (FDA) only allows food companies to say evidence "supports or promotes."

The FDA's definition of Medical Food is limited to products that provide crucial therapy for patients with inborn errors of metabolism, such as phenylketonuria (PKU). A Phenylalanine free food is an example of a Medical Food. Manufacturers markets "medical foods" such as low-protein spaghetti for chronic kidney disease (CKD). This 18 billion dollar industry is now very popular in Europe. In the USA, the marketing of gluten-free foods is all the rage! Medical foods are not drugs and they are not supplements. The FDA does not require formal approval of a medical food, but by law the ingredients must be "generally recognized as safe" (GRAS)

Be skeptical of supplements that claim to "support" or "boost."

More Groping through the Fog: Sell a Diet Book, Make a Fortune

There seems to be at least one diet book on the New York's Weekly Best Seller's List. These books are mostly about quick weight loss (look great at your High School Reunion, wedding, or in a swim suit).

Here are some of the most popular weight loss books, promising rapid and sustainable weight loss. As one book's miracle fades, another replaces it as hope springs eternal.

THE LIPID HYPOTHESIS

In 1904, the German scientist Felix Marchaud proposed the name "atherosclerosis" for an arterial disease characterized by obstructive patches, called plaques within arteries. These atheromatous arteries contained up to 20 times as much cholesterol as normal arteries.[17]

By 1912, Dr. James Herrick clearly identified and described how heart attacks are associated with atherosclerosis of the coronary arteries. That dietary saturated fats and cholesterol as found in animal protein could predictably increase a person's serum cholesterol was first established in the 1950's and 1960's. Much evidence now exists that an elevated serum concentration of cholesterol is a causal factor in the development of arterial atherosclerosis and coronary heart disease. Even a modest elevation to as little as 120mg low-density lipoproteins (LDL), also known as the "bad" cholesterol, can be significant in forming these obstructing plaques.

There are reputable scientists today that criticize this hypothesis because 100% evidence is not yet available. These nutritionists have not accepted the lipid hypothesis despite the growing body of evidence that supports it. Statements made publicly and widely disseminated by TV, radio, and the press have added to the confusion. The "cholesterol controversy" or more appropriately, the "saturated fat controversy," is being kept alive by special interest groups that are more concerned about the health of the beef, poultry, and dairy industries. Similar "controversy" over salt or sodium as a major cause of high blood pressure is now being disseminated by the major salt using, processed and frozen food industry.

Just as the tobacco industry has not succeeded in convincing intelligent adults that cigarettes are really harmless and non-addicting, those who suggest cholesterol, fats, or high salt intake are not related to heart disease and high blood pressure (hypertension) offer equally flimsy reasoning. Enough convincing evidence exists to strongly and safely recommend that, for continued good health, a diet should be low in saturated fats, cholesterol, simple sugars, and salt. It should contain moderate amounts of protein, be high in complex carbohydrates, fiber-rich foods and low in simple sugars.

In addition to saturated fats, trans fats, cholesterol, and sugar, there are other players that contribute to the development of atherosclerosis. There are genetic or familial factors, antioxidants, and possibly infectious agents, such as viruses or other microbes that may initially damage the lining of arterial walls, thus setting in motion the formation of cholesterol-laden atherosclerotic plaques. Particularly intriguing is the growing evidence pointing toward the role of germs or microorganisms—such as *Chlamydia pneumoniae,* herpes virus, and mycoplasma—in the causation of atherosclerosis and coronary artery disease.[18]

In the 1950's–1970's, heart disease was still believed to be caused primarily by stress. My father was told by his doctor to continue smoking because he was in a high stress business and "smoking reduces your stress!" Hard to believe now, but this was the dogma during the mid-20th century where physicians lined up to promote a favorite cigarette brand, "More doctors smoke Camels."

THE PRITIKEN DIET

Nathan Pritikin popularized his extremely low fat, high complex carbohydrate diet with claims that this diet could reverse atherosclerotic plaque and reverse the symptoms of type 2 diabetes mellitus. Pritikin suggested we eat whole, unprocessed, and natural carbohydrate-rich foods, such as grains and vegetables. Preferred foods include: Brown rice, millet, barley, oats, dark green, leafy vegetables, onions, potatoes, squash, beans, black turtle beans, chickpeas, lentils, pinto beans, apples, pears, strawberries, and bananas.

Some processed whole-grain foods, such as oatmeal, are on the plan. White flour pasta is permitted as long as it is with vegetables.

Small portions of lean beef, chicken, and low-fat dairy products. Fish: three servings per week of salmon or other fish rich in omega-3 fatty acids. Avoidance of any fried foods, dressing with fat, and fatty sauces. Eat three meals a day plus two snacks. Stay active and avoid salty foods. Artificial sweeteners are okay on the plan. He published his "Live Longer Now" that rationally explained, step-by-step, his interpretation of how the atheroma (plaque) developed within arterial walls. His nutrition program along with mild daily exercise, demonstrated the arrest of further development of arterial disease.

His hypothesis was rejected by the mainstream medical establishment.

As a pediatric resident, I was taught that hypertension, adult onset diabetes, and heart disease were the inevitable consequences of aging and stress. They were to be treated with the few medications that were available. Diet was seldom discussed. The idea that these diseases could be due to a high-fat diet further piqued my interest in nutrition. The sugar hypothesis was, in the meantime, "debunked" by corrupted but respected academics.

Dr. Dean Ornish's low fat diet is also based on vegetables, grains, and fruits. His reduced stress program for reversing heart disease is another major component and in many ways similar to the Pritikin Principle. It is a respected University of California-based program.[19]

HIGH FAT DIETS

THE ATKINS DIET

This diet is a low carbohydrate diet devised by Robert Atkins. The diet is carbohydrate restricted and in his book *Dr. Atkins' New Diet Revolution,* he argues that restricting carbohydrates is the "key" to weight loss. He states that the metabolic advantage of this diet is that "burning fat takes more calories so you expend more calories."[20] This explanation has not been shown to be valid. Nevertheless, the diet does curb the appetite and dieters were simply eating fewer calories. The initial weight loss was felt to be the result of increased water loss. Whether true or not, this diet lost popularity perhaps due to how boring it was and it did not appear to achieve durable weight loss.

THE KETOGENIC DIET: THE ULTIMATE LOW-CARB DIET

This diet is not something new. It has been used for almost 100 years to treat drug-resistant epilepsy in children. In the 1970's, Dr. Atkins popularized his very low carbohydrate diet for weight loss that began with a very strict two-week ketogenic phase. In essence, it is a diet that causes the body to release ketones into the bloodstream. Ketone bodies are molecules that arise from the metabolism of fatty acids and are converted into acetoacetate, beta-hydrozybutyrate, and acetone. What happens is a physiologic ketosis. Ketones in the blood are elevated and these compounds can function as an energy source for the body including the brain. Ketosis can be introduced during starvation, but also by carbohydrate restriction. This is referred to as nutritional ketosis. A low-carbohydrate, moderate-protein diet can lead to ketosis and is called a ketogenic diet. Most cells prefer to use blood sugar, which comes from carbohydrates as the body's main source of energy. In the absence of circulating blood sugar from food, the body starts to break down stored fat into these ketone molecules. As a result, there is weight loss, a major goal. However there may be other benefits such as lowering the A1C in diabetes.

Ketosis is well established as a treatment for epilepsy and is also effective in reducing harmful inflammation. Elevation of blood ketones have proved to be protective against tissue damage due to lack of oxygen, which occurs in severe respiratory infections, such as COVID-19. The hope is that the diet will reduce the systemic inflammation, known as a cytokine storm, that results in acute respiratory distress syndrome.

The possible effect on a range of neurological diseases, metabolic syndrome, cancer, and other conditions is currently under investigation.

The most common side effects of ketosis include headache, fatigue, dizziness, insomnia, exercise intolerance, constipation, and nausea, especially in the first days and weeks after starting a ketogenic diet. Breath may develop a sweet, fruity flavor via production of acetone that is exhaled because of its high volatility.[21]

Ketosis induced by a ketogenic diet should not be pursued by anyone with genetic disorders of fat metabolism or with pancreatitis because of the high dietary fat content.

THE MEDITERRANEAN DIET

Ancel Keys, a pioneer nutritionist, noticed that heart disease varied tremendously throughout the world. Finland had extremely high rates while Japan's rates were low until some Japanese moved to the United States and adopted a Western Diet. Those with the lowest rates of heart disease were from Crete. They ate quite a bit of fat, but mostly unsaturated fats such as those found in fish and olive oil. He promoted the Mediterranean diet. It was not a "no fat" diet. Dr. Keys recommended a diet of about 30% fat. It was one of substituting fats from highly saturated sources to one that was mostly monounsaturated and high in omega-3 essential fatty acids.

A recent study of the Mediterranean diet was published in the New England Journal of Medicine (NEJM 2/25/2013). In this trial that took place in Spain, researchers randomly assigned study volunteers at risk of heart disease to a Mediterranean or standard low-fat diet for five years, allowing the team to single out the effect of diet. Almost 7,500 older adults with diabetes or other heart risks were divided into one of three groups. Subjects continued the medications they had, such as statins or diabetic drugs. Two groups were instructed to eat a Mediterranean diet—one supplemented with extra-virgin olive oil and the other with nuts. The third study group ate a "control" diet, which emphasized low-fat dairy products, grains, fruits, and vegetables. Over the next five years, 288 study participants had a heart attack, stroke, or died from some type of cardiovascular disease. People on both Mediterranean diets were 28–30% less likely to develop cardiovascular disease than those on the general low-fat diet. This is the first randomized trial of any diet pattern to show benefit among people at risk, but initially without heart disease. Critics claim that this study has major design flaws.[22]

The Diet: It is a blend of Mediterranean diet components—not one particular ingredient—that promotes heart health.

A. Legumes, fresh vegetables, fruits as desserts, and cooking with olive oil
B. Fresh seafood and fish
C. Discouraging refined breads, pasta, sweets, sodas, red meats, and processed meats (salami, bologna, pepperoni, jerky)
D. Replacing a high-carbohydrate or high-saturated fat snack with a handful of nuts

E. Water or, for those adults, red wine with meals, instead of hard alcohol.

Although this was a high risk group, I see no reason that children should wait until they become high risk!

Ancel Keys died at the age of 101. His wife died when she was 97.

THE SOUTH BEACH DIET

The South Beach Diet is another weight-loss diet. It was popularized by cardiologist Arthur Agatston, and is a "low carb" diet such as the **Atkins Diet**. This diet does prohibit foods rich in simple carbohydrates such as white bread, white potatoes, and white rice. It does not require dieters to forgo carbohydrates entirely or even measure their intake. Instead, it focuses on the "glycemic impact" (short-term change in blood glucose) of foods. The South Beach Diet, named after a glamorous area of Miami, is higher in protein and monounsaturated fats but it's not a strict low-carb diet.

The stated purpose of the diet is to change the overall balance of the foods you eat to encourage weight loss and a healthy lifestyle.

Food sources of complex carbs, or so-called "good" carbs, include fruit, vegetables, whole grains, beans, and legumes. Simple carbs, or "bad" carbs, include sugar, syrup, and baked goods made from refined white flour.

If you severely restrict your carbohydrates, you may experience problems from ketosis. Ketosis occurs when you don't have enough sugar (glucose) for energy, so your body breaks down stored fat, causing ketones to build up in your body. Side effects from ketosis can include nausea, headache, mental fatigue, bad breath, and sometimes dehydration and dizziness.[23]

THE INFLAMMATION HYPOTHESIS

The hypothesis that inflammation is a core contributor to the development of heart disease and stroke is gaining more support as studies show this to be another major risk factor.

Inflammation may cause an atheroma (plaque) within the wall of an artery poised to explosively rupture through the artery wall. The body reacts by forming a blood clot and when this clot obstructs a heart artery, a heart attack is triggered. Plaque causing a clot from a diseased artery can travel to the brain, causing a stroke.

ESR and C-Reactive Protein (CPR)—inflammatory markers—are elevated in patients before, during, and after a heart attack or stroke. It has been observed that markers of inflammation, such as an elevated C-Reactive Protein, seems to be a predictor of future heart attack and is now routinely measured in adult patients along with other tests that measure inflammation.

Researchers continue to search for foods that promote inflammation, such as fatty acids, and microorganisms that might be triggers of acute heart attack. Influenza is a viral disease that is often underestimated. It is more than a slight "cold" and many heart attacks are followed by this illness due to the body's inflammatory response to viruses and bacteria. Most recently, the coronavirus that causes COVID-19 is another example of a virus that causes an inflammatory response.

"Free Radicals" are also suspected of causing inflammation and damage to the cellular lining of blood vessels. To prevent free radical damage, the body has a defense system of anti-oxidants. Anti-oxidants are molecules that can safely interact with free radicals and terminate the chain reaction before the arterial lining cells are damaged. The body can't manufacture the required vitamin antioxidants, such as Vitamin C, beta-carotene, Vitamin E, and lycopene. These must come from the diet (not pills!). Foods, such as blueberries, raspberries, blackberries, strawberries, and cranberries are excellent sources of antioxidants.

THE ZONE DIET

This diet, popularized by Dr. Barry Seals, aims to reduce cellular inflammation. To reach proper hormone balance he suggests fat consumption is essential for "burning" fat. He claims that the relatively high proportion of carbohydrates in low-fat/high-carbohydrate diets, compared with protein, increases the production of insulin, causing the body to store fat. When insulin levels are neither too high nor too low, then specific anti-inflammatory chemicals called eicosanoids are released. Sears claims that a 30:40 ratio of protein to carbohydrate triggers this effect. He calls this "the ZONE." Sears says that these natural anti-inflammatories are heart and health-friendly. No direct studies to verify his conclusions have been performed.

THE PALEOLITHIC DIET

Paleolithic nutrition refers to a "hunter gatherer" diet, first published by Walter L. Voegtlin in 1975 as the Stone Age Diet: Based on "in-depth" studies of Human Ecology and the Diet of Man. His thesis was that humans are carnivorous animals and our ancestor's diet was carnivorous— chiefly fats and protein with only small amounts of carbohydrates.

This diet has its roots in evolutionary biology. The charge is that our biochemistry and physiology are tuned to life conditions that existed some 10,000 years ago and that our bodies are genetically the same as they were at the end of the Paleolithic Era some 20,000 years ago. Proponents of this diet say that excessive consumption of the Western Diet and sedentary lifestyle contribute to many of the so-called diseases of civilization. There are no large or well-controlled studies to support this diet.

CONCLUSION

Which diet (I do not mean for weight loss when I use the term diet) is best?

The Atkins meat-based high fat plan? The Yudkin's very low sugar diet? The Pritikin plant based low fat plan? The low inflammatory diets? Or is it the Paleolithic Diet? Read on before you decide.

The above mentioned diets are either "weight loss" diets or diets designed to treat those who are sick, with heart disease, diabetes, gout, arthritis, metabolic syndrome, and the endless illnesses blamed on "old age."

Personally, I favor the Mediterranean Diet for children and adults. Do not confuse this with a high pasta and cheese diet. Olive oil is my favorite for cooking along with canola oil for baking. Although some olive oil enthusiasts suggest using a small amount of olive oil as a supplemental beverage, I do not. They belong to the, "more is better" school. The key is fresh vegetables, legumes, whole grains, unsalted nuts, poultry, fish, eggs, small amounts of very lean meats, and whole grains. Added sugar or juice and especially sugar-fat food combinations (as found in most "fast foods") should be avoided.

The Mediterranean "Diet" is not for losing weight. It is a diet for healthy living and designed to prevent many of the infirmities that blight those golden years.

This diet is mentioned here because it is the diet recently followed by former President Bill Clinton. It is a plant-based diet that excludes meats, eggs, poultry, and all dairy. In the "China Study," by Dr. T. Colin Campell, PhD, he recommends eating whole foods and not to rely on the idea that nutrient supplementation as the way to go.[24]

While on this diet, the president lived primarily on beans and other legumes, vegetables, and fruit, although on rare occasions he ate fish. Sorry, but he had to forego his favorite hamburgers and French fries after his heart attack.[25]

CHAPTER 3

Food Additives and Environmental Contaminants

A new policy statement from the American Academy of Pediatrics (AAP) reveals that more than 10,000 chemicals are permitted to be added to or have contact with foods.[26] Many of these are "generally regarded as safe" (GRAS) by the more recently highly politicized US Food and Drug Administration (FDA). In recent years the volume of chemicals used in food, "may contribute to disease and disability," according to the highly respected AAP.

Be aware of the fact that the Food Industry itself evaluated over 35% of GRAS classified chemicals with 64% being performed by expert panels appointed by manufacturers! The Food Industry should not be trusted on faith. This is one more example of the fox guarding the henhouse. I doubt that you or most readers or physicians are aware of this.

Researchers have specific health concerns over additives including chemical disrupters of endocrine system development, and phthalates, known to disrupt thyroid hormones, which are used as an antistatic agent in plastic packaging for foods.

There are perfluoroalkyl chemicals (PFC's) that are used in grease-proof paper and packaging and act as a thyroid disruptor as well as to reduce immune responses to vaccines. Then there are food colorings and additives such as nitrates, as stated earlier, common in processed meats.

The AAP recommends that you avoid microwaving foods and beverages in plastic, particularly infant formula and pumped breast milk and reduce the use of plastics in food storage.

I wish to add that exposure to these additives is especially found in low-income populations that may utilize prepared or processed foods at higher rates.

This is one more reason to consume fresh or frozen fruits and vegetables instead of fast and highly processed food.

SULFITE

Although the incidence of sulfite sensitivity is small in the general population, it can cause airway obstruction, cough, hives, and nasal congestion. The FDA banned the use of sulfites in fresh and raw fruit and vegetables in 1986. Commercial baby foods do not contain sulfites, but I do not recommend sulfite containing foods at any age, if they can be avoided. Certainly they should not be given to children with a history of hives or asthma. Sulfites are also commonly found in avocado dip, shrimp, shellfish, bacon, and cold cuts. Federal law requires food manufacturers to list the sulfite content of any product containing more than ten parts per million. The FDA has a "generally recognized as safe" list (GRAS) that can provide further information on sulfites.

HERBICIDES

ROUNDUP (GLYPHOSATE)

Used in yards, farms, and parks throughout the world, Roundup has long been a top-selling weed killer. But now researchers have found that one of Roundup's inert ingredients can kill human cells, particularly embryonic, placental, and umbilical cord cells.

The California Environmental Protection Agency's Office of Environmental Health Hazard Assessment confirmed that it would add glyphosate to California's Proposition 65 list of chemicals known to cause cancer. Monsanto sued to block the action but the case was dismissed. In a separate case, the court found that California could not require cancer warnings for products containing glyphosate. On June 12, 2018, the United States District Court for the Eastern District of California denied the California Attorney General's request for the court to reconsider the decision. The court found that California could only require commercial speech that disclosed "purely factual and uncontroversial information," and the science surrounding glyphosate carcinogenicity was not proven.

Claims have been made that glyphosate may be a cause of non-Hodgkins Lymphoma.[27]

CAVEAT EMPTOR!—BUYER BEWARE.

PHTHALATES

These chemicals are linked to lower fertility in men and ˅
are an endocrine disruptor. That is, they can interfere with est˷
tosterone, thyroid hormone, insulin, or other hormones, even at ˅
levels. Higher levels in pregnancy are linked to anatomical chang˷
infant boys and may affect their ability to father children in later life.

Phthalates may also affect fertility in women. Women with high levels of one particular phthalate reach menopause about four years earlier
than other women.

The FDA allows the use of 28 phthalates in food contact materials
and has not assessed their safety in more than 30 years.[28]

Consumer groups tested 30 cheese products, including boxed macaroni and cheese, for traces of phthalates. All but one of the 30 tested
positive. Sadly, I was not able to get the name of the one that was not
positive. We don't understand exactly how phthalates get into foods, but
this chemical is now ubiquitous. Phthalates are everywhere.

BISPHENOL A (BPA)

Another endocrine disrupter (it can act as an estrogenic compound)
is BPA. It is used to make a hard plastic, polycarbonate, and to protect
the insides of cans, jar lids, and bottle caps. It also is used to coat printed
receipts from cash registers, gas pumps, and ATM's. It is ubiquitous and
therefore nearly all of us have it in our bodies. We know that these chemicals correlate but do not establish a cause and effect proof in ADHD,
insulin resistance, and increased risk of diabetes type 2.[29]

Despite the emerging evidence suggesting that BPA may be harmful,
the FDA has ruled that it is safe. *Only use BPA free containers.*[30]

LEAD CONTAMINATION

Lead poisoning is a type of metal poisoning caused by lead in the
body. The brain is the most sensitive. Symptoms may include abdominal
pain, constipation, headaches, irritability, memory problems, inability to
have children, and tingling in the hands and feet.

Avoid using ceramic or glazed containers unless you are certain they
do not contain lead. Lead poisoning may result if lead leeches from these
bowls and contaminates the food.

(From Chris)

Ceramic salad bowls from Mexico or Central America often contain traces of lead. The vinegar in salad dressing may leech out traces of lead. Better to avoid such bowls for use and keep them as ornaments.

NITRATES AND NITRITES

Nitrates and nitrites are associated with processed meats and are potentially cancer-causing compounds. The Food Industry would like to have you believe that these preservatives may even be healthy! They ignore the fact that when nitrites are added to foods, such as lunch meats, and are consumed, they form a chemical called nitrosamine. Nitrosamines are carcinogenic or cancer producing. Once again, the propagandists of the corrupt Meat Food Industry takes this threat seriously and attacks the science by making light of it or even suggesting that these chemicals may be referred to as "health foods"! It reminds me of the tobacco industry's playbook.

Foods advertised as nitrate or nitrite "free" often contain nitrates or nitrites from hidden sources such as celery juice. Check the label of ingredients! Celery has a very high concentration of natural nitrate, and treating celery juice with a bacterial culture produces nitrite. The concentrated juice can then be used to produce "no nitrite added" processed meat. Curiously, regulations stipulate that the traditional curing process requires the addition of nitrite and thus "organic" processed meats that are treated with celery juice have to be labeled as "uncured." Pretty sneaky. Regardless of whether the nitrites come from celery juice or added nitrites, the outcome is the same, a high-sodium, high-saturated fat treat. You decide. I personally love hot dogs, but resist eating them too often.

PESTICIDES

The persons most at risk for pesticide poisoning are the field laborers using these chemicals. The degree of harm depends on the chemical and duration of exposure. Very small amounts of even the most toxic materials may do great harm. However, less-toxic materials in large amounts can also cause great harm. People, mostly farm laborers, are exposed to pesticides in three ways: breathing (inhalation exposure), oral exposure (getting it into the mouth), and skin or eyes exposure. Pesticides can enter the body by any one or all three of these routes.

Inhalation can happen if you breathe air containing a pesticide as a vapor, as an aerosol, or on small particles of dust. Oral exposure happens

STRAWBERRIES

when you eat food or drink water containing pesticides. Skin exposure causes irritation or burns, while, in more serious cases, your skin can absorb the pesticide into the body, causing other health effects. The more a person is exposed, the greater the chance of harm.

Children may be more sensitive to some pesticides than adults. Compared to adults, they breathe in more air and eat more food relative to their body size which increases their exposure. When they play on lawns or put objects in their mouths, they increase their chance of exposure to pesticides. Golf courses probably use the most pesticides and herbicides outside of farming.

CHLORPYRIFOS[31]

This pesticide belongs to the class of chemicals known as organophosphates. Organophosphates are poisonous (toxic) to nerve tissue. Acute poisoning can cause convulsions, respiratory paralysis, and, in extreme cases, death. If that is not enough, exposures during pregnancy to chlorpyrifos are associated with lower birth weight, reduced IQ, loss of working memory, attention disorders, and delayed motor development. It is so hazardous that the European Union (EU) has banned it. Chlorpyrifos was scheduled to be banned in California and New York. The Environmental Protection Agency (EPA) is an agency created to ensure that "no harm will result to infants and children from aggregate exposure" to pesticides. The EPA cannot take industry costs into consideration when protecting children from harmful pesticides. If the EPA cannot ensure that a pesticide won't harm children, the law is supposed to require the EPA to ban the use of the pesticide.[32]

A professor of mine would often warn me that "supposed to" has killed more people than the atom bomb!

On Feb. 6, 2020, Corteva, Inc (formerly Dow Chemical) announced it will stop selling the nerve agent pesticide chlorpyrifos, which is linked to brain damage in children. Corteva is the largest producer in the United States.[33]

Most of the reported acute cases of organophosphate poisoning are to farm workers and come from direct exposure during work. In response to the Farm Lobby, the Trump administration's EPA reversed the agency's own proposal and refused to ban chlorpyrifos![34]

WHY SHOULD I BUY ORGANIC PRODUCE?

Once a year an environmental group, The Environmental Working Group (EWG) publishes a list of fruit and vegetables with elevated levels of pesticides based on analysis of data from the U.S. Department of Agriculture (USDA). These are known as the "dirty dozen foods."[35]

THE 2020 DIRTY DOZEN FOOD LIST

- Strawberries
- Spinach
- Kale
- Nectarines
- Apples
- Grapes
- Peaches
- Cherries
- Pears
- Tomatoes
- Celery
- Potatoes

I encourage you to buy organic products as much as possible.

The USDA has developed strict rules and regulations to govern organic foods. Anything carrying the USDA organic seal can't be genetically engineered and also must be grown in soil that is free from prohibited substances such as synthetic fertilizers and pesticides.

Buying organic versions of the vegetables and fruits on the Dirty Dozen list might eliminate many possible risks associated with potential pesticide contamination. If fresh organic food is too expensive, frozen organic foods come at a much better price and last a long time. Plus, frozen organically produced food is typically picked and flash-frozen at its peak nutritional value. Most frozen produce may be more nutritious than fresh produce that has been sitting on a truck during transport to the supermarket and then sitting on the grocery shelves for days.

THE 2020 CLEAN FIFTEEN LIST

These conventionally raised produce items had the lowest amount of pesticide residues, with nearly all of them only containing four or fewer pesticides. Almost 70% of these samples had no pesticide residues whatsoever:

- Avocados
- Sweet corn
- Pineapple
- Onions
- Papaya
- Sweet Peas (Frozen)
- Eggplant
- Asparagus
- Cauliflower
- Cantaloupes
- Broccoli
- Mushrooms
- Cabbage
- Honeydew Melon
- Kiwi

Eating enough produce is the most important thing, regardless of whether it is organic or conventionally grown. The Dirty Dozen list must not deter you from eating produce even if it isn't organic because the nutritional benefits of fruit and vegetables are still there and the vitamins, minerals, and antioxidants provided from produce are essential.

You can minimize the effects of pesticides by washing your food right.

WASH YOUR FOOD AND WASH IT RIGHT

Wash all your fruits and vegetables. The U.S. Food and Drug Administration suggests washing them to remove most of the contact pesticide residues that normally appear on the surface of the vegetables and fruits.[36]

Just using cold water removes 75–80% of pesticide residues.

Another recommended method is the vinegar soak. A mixture of 10% vinegar and 90% tap cold tap water also works. Soak your veggies and fruits in them, stir, and then rinse thoroughly with cold water.

Be careful while washing fruits like berries and those with a thin peel as the solution might damage their outer porous skin.

See fda.gov/consumers/consumer-updates/7-tips-cleaning-fruits -vegetables for more information on how to wash fruits and vegetables.

CHAPTER 4

Feed Your Body Right from Birth to Adulthood

FEEDING YOUR INFANT

First of all, it is a must for every mother to pay special attention to what she eats beginning with the first moments she becomes aware that she is pregnant. If it is a planned pregnancy, she should begin well before trying to become pregnant. The foods that a mother eats during pregnancy affect the health of the baby. That means avoiding foods high in mercury and starting a multivitamin mineral preparation containing extra iron and folic acid. In addition, it is especially important to stop smoking. Discuss with your physician whether it is safe to continue with medicines you were prescribed, over-the-counter medications and herbals. Be aware of your water supply. If it is well water, *get it tested*. Test your home's water for lead or, if you use well water, check it for nitrites from soil contamination. If you live where there is known lead contamination, as was found in cities such as Flint, Michigan or Newark, New Jersey, this is especially important.

Eating fish is important, but avoid the fish that have the highest level of mercury such as shark, swordfish, king mackerel, and tilefish. Check local advisories about the safety of fish caught in your local lakes, rivers, and coastal areas. Pregnant moms should include fish that are generally lower in mercury. These include shrimp, scallop, canned light tuna, salmon, pollack, catfish, sole, flounder, butterfish, cod, fresh water trout, lobster, clams, tilapia, and red snapper. Mercury is a metal that occurs naturally in the environment and is increased by industrial pollution. Most people are not affected by tiny amounts of mercury. If a woman is exposed to high levels of mercury before or while she is pregnant, her health and the baby's health are threatened. Babies exposed to mercury in the womb can suffer severe nervous system damage, brain damage, learning disabilities, and hearing loss.[37]

Limit your consumption of fish to three 12 oz servings of fish per week to avoid the harmful effects of mercury, but don't give up fish. It is an important part of the diet!

Eat fish that is high in DHA (docosahexaenoic acid, an omega-3 fatty acid) such as salmon; low- or non-fat dairy and calcium rich foods; legumes, such as black beans or kidney beans; brown rice; fruit rich in antioxidants and Vitamin C such as citrus fruit, organic strawberries, and organic blueberries; whole grain breads and cereals low in added sugar; and especially leafy greens. Eat iron-rich or iron-fortified foods plus foods such as lean meats or meat alternatives.

Drink sufficient water. The amount varies tremendously because it depends on your diet. Pay attention to thirst. The color of your urine should be light yellow.

Avoid some of my old favorite foods such as salami, hot dogs, and lunch meats. They are high in sodium (salt), nitrite, and are a big No-No!

What other foods are completely off-limits during pregnancy?

Raw or undercooked meat, including beef, poultry and pork.

Raw fish, especially shellfish, sashimi, and sushi.

Soft scrambled eggs.

Raw sprouts, especially alfalfa sprouts[38]

ALCOHOL CONSUMPTION

Of special danger is the consumption of alcohol. The Fetal Alcohol Spectrum Disorders (FASDs) are a group of conditions found in children of mothers who consumed alcohol while pregnant. The condition may cause physical, mental, behavioral, or learning disabilities. Although the worst cases in my pediatric practice were in infants and children adopted from countries such as Russia, Rumania, and other countries where the culture of high-alcohol consumption is pervasive. Too many infants were born in Marin County, California and the USA with the Fetal Alcohol Spectrum Disorder.

No amount of alcohol should be considered safe.

For more information, visit the National Organization on Fetal Alcohol Syndrome (NOFAS): nofas.org/about-fasd.

CHAPTER 5

Breastfeeding

Breastfeeding provides the best nutrition for an infant. The practice is gaining in popularity again as more information is reaching parents. Breast milk is truly a magic food, and your breast milk is unique to your baby. It is more variable and valuable than what is suggested in scientific tables found in standard nutrition books.

Diet affects the composition of breast milk. A vegetarian's breast milk is different in fatty acid pattern from that of a non-vegetarian. Breast milk also changes depending on the age of the baby—the breast milk produced by the mother of a preterm infant is more suited to the needs of her baby and is not the same as the milk from the mother of a full-term infant. At nine months of age the breastfed baby is receiving milk which is different from the milk received at one week. Depending on what mother eats, the milk may taste different from day to day, compelling the infant to adapt to new tastes. This prepares your baby's palate for when you introduce semisolid foods. Milk expressed in the first few minutes of breastfeeding, called foremilk, has a lower fat content than hind or later milk. That is one important reason why many infants need to nurse longer than a few minutes at a time. One mother may breastfeed briefly a few times a day and the baby rapidly gains weight while another mother may have to breastfeed two to three times as long and more often to provide as many calories to her infant. If your infant breastfeeds less than the time "suggested" by your "how to breastfeed" books, and your baby is thriving, don't fret! Breast milk varies tremendously from mother to mother.

Breast milk is high in saturated fats and cholesterol and there is good reason for this. Many parents look at the listed ingredients on a can of infant formula and wonder why it contains so much saturated fat, cholesterol, and sugar, since they may have been have been told repeatedly that fats, cholesterol, and sugar should be avoided in their diets. Babies are different. They are not merely small adults! Babies need saturated fat, cholesterol, and milk-sugar. Ample amounts of these nutrients are essential in these early months because of the baby's high energy needs and rapid growth of the brain and nervous system. Infant nutrition becomes even more complicated because the amount and types of unsaturated fat and fatty acids found in breast milk are different from what is found in other milks such as cow or goat milk. This is one of the reasons it is so important for parents to have some understanding of the more complex nutritional needs of children and to respect the possibility that there are probably many more nutritional unknowns to be discovered.

Although breast milk contains a lot of fat, it must be absorbed by the baby to do any good. Lipase is an enzyme which digests fat; it comes primarily from the pancreas. At birth and for the first few weeks of life, pancreatic lipase is in short supply, possibly due to the immaturity of the pancreas. Pancreatic lipase can't be given by mouth to correct this deficiency because it would be destroyed by the stomach acid before reaching the intestine. However, breast milk contains a lipase which resists stomach acid and which aids pancreatic lipase in the digestive process. Neither cow nor goat milk contains this unique enzyme. It is possible that this extra lipase helps breastfed infants to absorb more fat. Another lipase, called lingual lipase, comes from the base of the infant's tongue and is produced in response to sucking. This may help to explain why babies, particularly in the first few months of life, want to continue sucking even after they have finished breastfeeding . This "non-nutritive sucking" has been used as a rational justification for offering a pacifier to a newly-born infant.

I am not against pacifiers, but believe they should be postponed until breastfeeding is established, thus avoiding "nipple confusion," and initial birth weight is regained. Nursery nurses often promote the pacifier because it calms the hungry infant. It is used in the noble spirit of letting the tired or often exhausted mother get some needed rest. What is not appreciated is that as a consequence of this, the mother's breasts are not stimulated sufficiently, and as a result there is often a delay in milk production. The seemingly benign and benevolent act of giving the pacifier (or bottles of water) during the few days following birth is often responsible for nursing failure. Please refrain from the temptation of using a pacifier until your milk production is enough for your infant to achieve adequate weight gain. This does not mean that you should allow the infant to become dehydrated. Give water but use an eyedropper instead of a nipple or a sucking device so you don't confuse the infant. Nipple confusion is a common issue and often results in "breastfeeding failure."

Infant's sucking on a breast stimulates jaw development and therefore this should be encouraged when possible instead of putting pumped breast milk in a bottle.

When a mother doesn't want to breastfeed, or can't, the second choice is a store bought formula of cow-milk base, or sometimes an "elemental formula." Ideally, your baby's doctor should prescribe the specific formula, technique of preparation, and appropriate schedule for bottle feeding. These directions should be based on your baby's own nutritional and digestive needs.

VITAMINS FOUND IN BREAST MILK

A look at the vitamin content of breast milk and formula reveals some interesting comparisons. Both human and cow milk are rich in Vitamin A and Vitamin B complex. Cow milk is low in Vitamin C. For this reason, babies fed cow milk alone need supplements. Well-nourished mothers produce milk sufficient in Vitamin C.

Cow milk has no Vitamin D. Because of this, rickets, a disease of children characterized by softening of the bones as a result of lack of Vitamin D, was a common occurrence in the past and still is in countries where milk is not fortified with Vitamin D3. This vitamin may also be in low supply in breast milk. Vitamin supplements therefore are a good idea for babies, especially those who get little sunlight. There will be more information on how sunshine helps the body manufacture Vitamin D in the section devoted to vitamins & minerals.

Another vitamin that is low in human milk but needed for blood clotting is Vitamin K. Breastfed infants are prone to a bleeding disease which in rare cases results in sometimes fatal bleeding into the brain. Fortunately, this can be prevented by giving the infant Vitamin K, either by mouth or by shot. Vitamin K is now given by a nurse to almost all infants shortly after birth. Cow milk formulas are fortified with extra Vitamin K so babies on formula are actually less susceptible to this disease than those who are breastfed. The breastfed infant remains low in Vitamin K the first 8 days of life. Religious Jews delay circumcising their son until he is 8 days old. This is the time it takes bacteria in the intestines to produce sufficient Vitamin K. It is this Vitamin K that is needed to prevent prolonged bleeding after circumcision as well as a catastrophic bleed into the infant's brain, a rare but preventible event.[39]

Vitamin E is found in greater amounts in human milk than in cow milk. Skimmed cow milk contains no Vitamin E. Infants fed only non-fat milk develop what is called "failure to thrive," infections, extremely dry skin, and blood problems.

Besides the immune factors, growth, and brain development factors found in breast milk, I am certain it contains many other yet undiscovered nutritional factors that nature created during our evolution. I strongly suggest that mothers continue to breastfeed for at least six months whenever possible, or better yet, up to one year.

THE ART OF BREASTFEEDING

It is the art of breastfeeding rather than the chemistry of breast milk that is of importance right away to a new mother. The nurturing aspect of breastfeeding has a potent emotional effect upon the bond between infant and mother. Unfortunately, there are a lot of worries around breastfeeding, and many myths exist. Therefore, the aid of a well-trained helper is the most important first step in breastfeeding. Beware of the helper who suggests pacifiers, sugar water, or putting the infant on an "every 2–3 hour schedule" the first week of life. This advice usually leads to insufficient sucking, which in turn leads to a delay in milk production, and ultimately leads to a frustrated exhausted mother who turns to a formula. At that moment, the infant gobbles down the formula and the mother concludes that the infant has chosen not to breastfeed. Often, the physician agrees and thus pays only lip service to supporting breastfeeding. There is now a group of specialist nurses, "Certified Lactation Consultants," who truly understand the art and science of breastfeeding. I recommend that one be consulted before the day of your infant's birth. Different opinions and techniques can be very confusing to the new mother. A breastfeeding specialist, along with your pediatrician, can help you establish a plan for the early weeks of breastfeeding that is specific to your baby's needs and breastfeeding style.

Recently, "tongue tie" is used as a diagnosis to blame nursing failure. I believe this condition is too loosely used to explain why some infants have difficulty latching on to a mother's nipple.[40]

Breastfeeding failure is a rare event in Denmark where over 95% of women breastfeed their infants. What do they know that Americans don't?

HINTS TO PREVENT TENDER BREASTS

1. Use a hair dryer to blow-dry your breast for about 20–30 seconds after each breastfeeding. This is very soothing and helps tender breasts to heal.

2. Be sure the infant takes more than the tip of the nipple into its mouth. Remove the infant from the breast by first breaking the suction with your finger.

3. Correct position is critical. Call a lactation specialist immediately if you even think you might be having any breastfeeding problem. Do not delay. Small problems are easier to solve than big ones.

4. Don't allow yourself to become frustrated. Some infants are not very interested in breastfeeding the first 24–36 hours , especially after a cesarean section. Ask your lactation helper whether an electric (Medela) breast pump is needed.

5. Fatigue and poor nutrition are enemies to good breastfeeding. Rest and good eating are essential. This is not the time to go on a crash diet. A new mom needs a helper at home. She doesn't need a nurse! The helper should take care of running the home, the cleaning, shopping, preparing food, laundry, and giving that two-year-old sibling some special attention. If daddy or grandma is not an option, enlist a relative or close friend to help. If your budget can afford it, hire a helper. The feeling of isolation and facing the responsibility of running a household in addition to caring for an infant is often overwhelming and has a profoundly negative effect upon successful breastfeeding.

6. A nipple shield (Medela brand) may be needed for inverted nipples, as well as a high quality electric breast pump. Consult a lactation specialist at least one month before the delivery of your baby if you have inverted nipples or if you are not certain. (Your baby might come early, so find help in advance.) There are many things that can be done early to keep this from becoming a problem. The lactation specialist may suggest devices that can be worn under the bra and over the nipple during the month prior to delivery. She will let you know, after examining your breasts, if you need them.

There are many excellent books to be found on breastfeeding. A classic is, "The Womanly Art of Breastfeeding" as well as "The Breastfeeding Mother's Guide to Making More Milk." I highly recommend both.

Formula Feeding

Formulas should be reserved for those who truly can't breastfeed or for those who choose not to breastfeed only after being taught about the nutritional advantages of breast milk. The final decision for or against breastfeeding should rest with the mother. In the meantime, don't think breastfeeding is another fad. It has been tested for thousands of years and has followed the evolution of our species.

WHAT IS THE DIFFERENCE BETWEEN BREAST MILK VS COW MILK FORMULA?

The salt content of breast milk is only 150mg per liter, whereas cow milk contains 500mg per liter or over three times as much salt. It is unknown whether this extra salt intake from cow milk could set a baby up for high blood pressure later in life, but this remains a worrisome consideration. About 15% of infants are believed to be salt sensitive.[41] This is one area of research that desperately needs to be studied by a major university, and not corrupted by or subsidized by the Food Industry. In the meantime, with lack of scientific proof to guide us, the low salt content of breast milk should be our model. I trust nature's model better than the Food Industry or nutritionists who used to suggest salt may not be a bad addition to an infant's or child's diet! (Do not use the Salt Industry's research as a guide!) Salt is now forbidden by law to be added to some "baby food." Recently the sodium content of formula has been lowered by manufacturers to approximate breast milk.

Parents are led to believe that lots of minerals and calcium are good for young children, but cow and goat milk have a much greater mineral content than human milk, and this could harm an infant. The high calcium content in cow milk, (1200mg vs. 300 mg in breast milk!) is too great a load on the infant's immature kidneys and should be avoided until the baby is over 12 months old. Another reason to avoid whole cow milk during the first year of life is its high-phosphorus content—six times that of human milk. In rare cases, such a high-phosphorus content can drop calcium levels in the blood, causing newborns to have seizures.

The iron content of breast milk may appear to be tiny at only 0.5mg per 100ml. However, almost 50% of this iron is absorbed, making it the most usable iron available. Cow milk contains nearly the same amount of iron but, by contrast, only 10% is absorbed. Infants who drink cow milk often become iron deficient by 10 months! For this reason most cow milk formula is fortified with 12–18mgs of iron per liter. Contrary to popular myth, this added iron will not lead to iron overload, bowel discomfort, spitting up, colic, or constipation. Premature infants may have diminished stores of iron and additional iron supplementation may be recommended by your pediatrician or healthcare provider.

Trace elements found in breast milk are different in type and concentration compared with cow or goat milk. As an example, there is less zinc in human milk than in cow milk, but a baby can use almost 60% of it. Only about 45% of zinc present in cow milk, although higher in milligrams, is available for use. Adequate zinc is needed to enhance infant growth. Also, a baby who gets too little zinc may be very cranky or suffer from an eczema-like rash on hands, feet, face, and the genital region. That is why zinc is added to commercial formulas to correct for this deficiency.

HERE ARE A FEW MORE BOTTLE FEEDING TIPS

1. Select a nipple that is available in most drug stores. Infants become attached to the nipple they are started on and often refuse to use another type. I can recall horror stories from parents who were up all night going from one pharmacy to another searching for the only type nipple their infant would take.

2. Select a bottle that is Bisphenol A (BPA) free. The plastic bag type bottles, such as Playtex, do not prevent air swallowing. Infants swallow air regardless of the bottle type and this is normal. Colic or gassiness is not prevented by a Playtex type of bottle.

3. Bottles do not need to be boiled or sterilized. They can be cycled through the dishwasher or washed and rinsed well by hand using a bottle-brush. Extra rinsing is important in order to remove all residual detergent.

4. Boiling nipples will destroy them. Wash them thoroughly by hand with soap and water and allow the nipples to air dry in a clean cup or bowl.

5. Both glass or plastic bottles are okay as long as they do not contain BPA or other endocrine disruptors. I prefer the BPA free plastic ones since they won't break when the baby throws one across the room. (See Chapter Three for more information on pesicides, etc.)

6. Do not warm bottles in the microwave. Warming of the bottle's contents is uneven and the formula or expressed breastmilk continues to cook for about a minute after removing the container from the microwave. An infant's tongue and mouth could easily be scalded by a bottle heated this way.

GOAT MILK

Goat milk is low in folic acid (folate), and because of this infants fed only goat milk often develop a severe anemia called megaloblastic anemia. Goat milk has achieved fad status in some circles because of its falsely supposed likeness to breast milk. Parents who are concerned about their infant's slow weight gain, irritability, or frequent infections, are tempted to try goat milk as a remedy. But for reasons pointed out above, it is better to defer offering goat milk during the first year. Before making such a change, discuss this with your doctor.

CHAPTER 7

Colic

Pediatricians are as susceptible to non-scientific behavior as the rest of us. When faced with a colicky infant, they often act in such a manner as he or she first selects and later switches infant formulas. Since many infants are irritable or colicky beginning at two weeks of age through three-and-a-half months of life, a ritual of formula changing often begins when the baby is about ten days old. By that time the desperate calls begin with predictable regularity. Instead of carefully explaining the nature of colic, the physician often elects to take the shortcut and changes the formula. This usually keeps the telephone quiet for another 2–3 days! Another culprit, called "reflux" is then postulated and a stomach acid suppressing drug may be prescribed.

What happened to me when I cared for my oldest daughter is typical. At the time I was in my third year of medical school and I was about to learn my first practical lesson in pediatrics. She was breastfed for 4–6 weeks, which was considered a long time. In those years most infants were bottle fed. If the mother breastfed, it was rare to continue beyond three months. My daughter was a skinny and irritable infant. Her knees were always red because they were in constant motion. She cried often, starting at ten days of age, and with such persistence, at first in the middle of the night, and later beginning at 4–5 p.m., that we were asked to move from our apartment because the neighbors couldn't stand the noise!

Later, even hours after breastfeeding or taking her formula, she would spit up. Our pediatrician suggested that my wife stop eating dairy, chocolate, "gassy vegetables," and spicy foods. For a couple of days we thought our daughter was improving, but by the weekend she was back at it. Like clockwork, as soon as I came home at around 5 p.m. she started crying and fussing until after midnight. We were then instructed to try another formula. But our daughter continued to draw up her legs, turn red, and cry, pass gas, and cry again. Next a soy formula was suggested. "This may be easier to digest," he explained. The colic continued. Another brand of soy formula was then recommended with similar disappointment. Maybe she's constipated, I reasoned. The elderly lady down the hall suggested a "suppository" or inserting the "end of a thermometer." We were willing to try almost anything and did this unhealthy maneuver for a few days. At first I thought we were on to a cure, but it soon became clear that the relief was not long lasting. "Perhaps the baby can't handle the iron in the formula," was the next week's telephoned advice. I later learned there was about as much iron in the soy formula he recommended as was in the last formula. The spitting and crying persisted after what I thought might have been a one or two day reprieve. The next suggestion seemed to help the most. Our doctor showed us how to swaddle her, and this did have some calming effect. He also suggested that we have her sleep in her infant seat to prevent "reflux," and prescribed an antacid and anti-gas drops. In those days gasoline was cheap, so I would buckle her in her car seat and drive around the block for an hour. Another popular method was to put the infant in a seat on the dryer. This motion has a calming effect. I promised the landlady I'd do this nightly, but she still asked us to leave our second apartment. We had three different apartments that first year of our daughter's life.

With all the scientific progress we have made over the past decade, no treatment surpasses holding and walking a colicky infant. There is little evidence that changing formulas or putting a breastfeeding mother on a "dairy-free, non-gassy, or non-spicy food" diet helps colic, but such advice continues to be freely prescribed. For the past few years, prescribing colicky infants anti-reflux medication had become another popular non-evidence based practice.

Nobody has yet determined, with certainty, the cause of colic. This periodic fussiness appears at about two weeks of age and often persists to three and a half months. Colic peaks around six weeks of age and then gradually becomes less intense. Most infants have a daily "fussy" period between 5 p.m. and 11 p.m. During this time the infant cries, turns red in the face, draws up his or her legs, passes gas, and appears to be in pain. The source of the pain is unclear, but most parents believe the pain arises in the gastrointestinal tract and therefore calls it a bellyache or thinks it is constipation. For this reason parents blame the pain on diet, if it is a breastfed baby, or the formula, in formula-fed infants. There is little proof that milk formula, with or without iron, is the culprit. Nevertheless changing formulas is the traditional advice, if for no other reason than to "buy time" until the infant is over three months old. Then miraculously the baby is able to tolerate breast milk even if the mother eats beans, cabbage, or drinks cow milk. The formula-fed infant now tolerates formulas that were stopped earlier. The scientific community doubts that allergy to milk or lactose intolerance is often the cause of this periodic fussiness or "colic." Nothing better than walking your infant during these hours has been invented, but swings, music, vibrating beds, and other devices have been helpful. Many medicines have been tried. Sometimes they seem to work, but the placebo effect may be the cause of temporary improvement. There are a host of other things that can be done to help parents through this stressful period. Be sure to let your pediatrician know if your child has symptoms of colic.

CHAPTER 8

First Foods

The timing of the introduction of semi-solid foods to infants is confusing to parents and physicians alike. As a pediatrician in training, I was taught to have infants avoid dairy until 1 year of age, eggs until 2 years, peanuts, tree nuts, and seafood until 3 years. At 4 to 6 months, the baby may require more calories than breastfeeding provides, and you may decide to introduce semi-solid foods (often referred to as, "complementary" food). Most of this information would have been equally valid if it were coming from my grandmother. The "baby food industry" has jumped in with Madison Avenue recommendations labeled as "first foods, then second foods," etc. More recently the Academy of Pediatrics has attempted to be more "scientific" in the recommendation for the timing and type of foods.

HONEY

Another food to be avoided until the baby is over one year, (although not an allergen) is honey, as it has been linked to infant botulism.[42,43] Botulism causes muscle weakness in infancy, often beginning with facial weakness, droopy eyelids, or the loss of ability to sit. Constipation is another early sign of infant botulism. If not treated early it can cause paralysis of the muscles of breathing. Although this is a rare condition, should you ever suspect it in your infant, call your physician immediately and tell him or her of your concern.

For many years I have worked in multiple countries and continents with families and observed, at first in horror, what mothers of different cultures fed their infants and children. Babies were breastfed for months and fed the same foods that were eaten by the family, without fear of food allergy. When questioned, they laughed at me, and, fortunately, ignored my advice. When I suggested anaphylaxis from introducing fish too early they just rolled their eyes! Mothers would eat and chew nuts and then give it to their infant. Could it be that they knew more about infant feeding than I, a highly-trained pediatrician? As it turns out, the answer is yes!

Our son married a woman who grew up in Beijing, China. Their daughter was fed the traditional diet of her Chinese mother. My son could not believe what she was fed, and what she loves to eat from the Chinese market. At an early age she would try anything and still enjoys almost any food. This was a positive change from my son, who was and remains a picky eater. My Vietnamese patients often feed fish soup to their infants beginning at 4–5 months of age. This is a cultural practice, and it is common for different cultures to follow a traditional approach to infant feeding. For example, the Indian infant who is often fed by the grandmother, gets what was given to her as an infant. With success!

Many people believe that introducing semi-solid food at two to three months, especially at the last feeding of the evening, will cause an infant to sleep through the night. After all, it seems logical that the increase in bulk will keep the baby full longer. Unfortunately careful studies show that semi-solid foods in the diet have no or minimal effect on the age at which an infant begins to sleep through the night.

Because the rapidly growing infant needs iron to build muscle and red blood cells, I recommend an iron-fortified cereal such as baby brown rice and oatmeal cereal. On a practical level, these commercially available dry cereals are a convenient way to get your baby used to taking semi-solid foods by spoon. Infants fed iron-fortified commercial formula usually get sufficient iron from this source; however, iron rich foods are needed the first year and beyond to fulfill the needs of a rapidly growing infant, especially if the infant was born prematurely.

Eating habits begin early, so I strongly encourage parents to introduce nutritionally important foods early. Don't be afraid to introduce other cereals, such as barley, rye, and wheat. These are recommendations that are best described as traditional, and not evidence based. Avoid putting cereal or foods in a bottle as it delays a baby's adjustment to textures. Some parents do this and go on with chores. Instead, hold or attend your infant during feedings. Your baby needs this attention and social contact. After all, feeding an infant is more than nutrition. If you are too busy to feed food to your infant, delay the semi-solid part of the feeding until you have time to relax and nurture your baby. Enjoy the baby during this special period in his or her life. It goes by quickly!

Feeding the infant may also afford the father a chance to bond with his baby. This should not be interpreted to mean that fathers need to feed their baby to fall in love with them. We know that many fathers fall in love with their baby without ever feeding them. (We refer to this as, "bonding.")

Experiment with textures, first by adding breast milk or formula to the dry cereal to make a thin gruel and then gradually make it thicker if the infant tolerates it without gagging. I'm not aware of any scientific studies that examine the long term consequences of early versus later exposure to different tastes or textures. One good reason for starting semi-solids in the first place, is to give the non-breast fed baby a variety of foods as a safeguard against the nutritional unknowns.

The caveat, "Eat a variety of foods," is difficult to follow if your only food source is breast milk or formula. Fortunately, breast milk is a near perfect food for infants. If an infant's total diet is commercial formula, a vital nutrient may be missing. So until we learn a lot more about how to make a perfect formula, it may be wise to add a variety of semi-solid foods to an infant's diet beginning at four to six months of age or even earlier.

Many parents want to know exactly how many teaspoons of food to give their child and wonder how to tell whether the baby is getting enough or too much. The answers you will find in most baby books are intentionally vague. That is because babies vary so much in their specific needs. All those charts and calorie formulas are guidelines that are seldom necessary to use. Look at your child. Is he or she too thin? Then offer more food or increase the frequency of feedings. Too plump? Then decrease amounts a little. If you are uncertain, the safest thing is to discuss this important issue with your pediatrician or healthcare provider during a "well child" checkup where the baby can be weighed, measured, and observed in person.

Don't believe that a fat baby is healthier than a slender infant. Many breastfed infants are slender, and this may be normal, especially among certain ethnic groups. A fat infant may become a fat adult. If obesity runs in your family, be especially careful not to overfeed your infant. The myth that breastfed infants are protected from obesity later in life is not supported by evidence.

A Word about Food Allergies

WHEAT, MILK, AND OTHER FOOD INTOLERANCES

The BIG 8. Approximately 90% of food allergy reactions occur from one of eight common foods in the United States called "The Big 8." These foods include: milk, eggs, peanuts, tree nuts, fish, crustaceans, shellfish, wheat, and soy.

My granddaughter was diagnosed with "acid reflux" as a cause of her persistent bellyaches, headaches, and stress, because she seldom smiled and moved as if she had a dark cloud following her. She was a twin, and her brother was a happy, mischievous kid who was many inches taller than she. Finally, she was referred to the university hospital and was found to have severe celiac disease. The treatment is a lifelong gluten-free diet. Her response to this diet was almost immediate. She began to smile, enjoy her life, grew several inches, and revealed her gifted nature.

Because we now have a simple blood test to determine whether a child's belly pains are due to celiac disease, an entire industry has developed providing "gluten-free" foods. This has made my granddaughter's life much easier. She will be graduating college soon and is leading a pain-free young adulthood with a major in engineering.

WHEN TO BEGIN FRUIT AND VEGETABLES

Another common recommendation is to start fruit before vegetables. There is little scientific information to support what order is best. Pediatricians do almost as well as grandmothers when it comes to choosing first foods. Almost all schedules are speculative, intuitive, or anecdotal. The message is, You decide!

Apples and pears are popular fruits, and most babies tolerate them quite well. Cooked carrots, squash, yams, and potatoes are foods I personally recommend to my patients. If these are tolerated, I suggest adding peas, strained spinach, beets, beans, broccoli, and brussels sprouts. However, I'm not dogmatic about the order in which foods are introduced. The choice is yours. That's part of the fun of being a parent.

I have more concern about the practice of adding a little salt or sugar to the baby's food, whether done by the commercial baby food company or the parent. In Europe, Asia, Africa, Central and South America, parents introduce soups at an early age. They put all these vegetables in a broth and mash or blend it into a soup. Infants usually love this and as the baby matures, the soup takes on a more lumpy, stew-like texture. To avoid giving your child too much salt or sugar, use a non-salted broth and forget the pinch of salt that makes it tasty to your palate!

Experiment with textures. Some babies without teeth may gum lumpy food easily, while other infants with teeth may gag on the same foods. As the baby matures, more and more textures can be tolerated until eating "grown-up" food cut in small pieces will be eaten.

When foods aren't pureed, you may notice partially digested material in the bowel movement and is quite normal. Stool color also changes with different foods. Don't be alarmed if the bowel movement is green. The only colors of concern in B.M.s are red, jet black, or cream-clay. Red and black may suggest bowel bleeding, while the clay color may be associated with a liver problem. However, colors often reflect the color of the foods eaten such as beets, peas, or spinach. Spinach, by the way, is an excellent natural laxative for infants as well as adults. It is not, however, the fabulous source of iron it's reputed to be. The baby doesn't absorb the iron in spinach as well as many other iron-rich foods.

PROTEIN AND YOUR INFANT

Today, health-conscious parents who know that meat, fish, or chicken are good sources of protein, wonder if they shouldn't be providing those foods to their baby. They often think of milk as a "calcium" food and forget that it is also very rich in protein. In fact, a 13-pound infant requires only 12–13 grams of protein daily, which is easily provided by breastfeeding or feeding three eight-ounce bottles of formula a day. The reason for suggesting the introduction of the above foods is not necessarily because of their protein content, but because they are an excellent source of the much needed mineral iron. There is little clinical evidence against beginning meats as a first food. It's your baby, so you decide what the first foods will be! The fatty acids, ARA and DHA (see "Nutrition 101" for more in depth details) are also found in fish and are important in eye and brain development. My mother used to tell me that fish was a "brain food" and encouraged me to eat it as a young child. Now it appears that she may have been correct. But remember, fish is a potent allergen, so consult with your healthcare provider before introducing it.

After one year of age, when the baby switches to cow milk, more protein will be provided than mother's milk or formula. In fact, three 8 oz. cups or bottles of cow milk a day contain enough protein for infants up to 30 pounds. So there's really no need to worry about insufficient protein. Because cow milk is iron-poor, it's important to introduce iron-rich foods, as explained earlier, and to make vegetables a significant part of the daily diet. I don't recommend ham, bacon, sausage, hot dogs, or lunch meats because of their high salt, saturated fat, and nitrite content. There are better choices to obtain important nutrients than from these "holiday foods."

Partially cooked meats are dangerous. Thorough cooking is needed to kill contaminating bacteria or parasites that can cause deadly diarrhea such as E. coli, salmonella-shigella, and campylobacter, as well as the diseases toxoplasmosis, trichinosis, or tapeworms.

Some nutritionists recommend beef or chicken liver as a good source of iron and vitamins. It is true that liver contains many important nutrients, but I no longer recommend liver as a nutritional source. As a detoxifying organ, the liver may contain a high concentration of all sorts of environmental poisons. There are safer ways to obtain these nutrients. I don't feel good about feeding liver to infants or children, and that includes the popular liverwurst sandwich.

OTHER CAUTIONARY NOTES

Plain pasteurized yogurt, Greek yogurt, and cottage cheese are fine foods (unless filled with added sugar as in Yoplait and some "fruit" Greek or non-fat yogurts), but since your less than one-year old infant is already consuming a lot of milk, he or she doesn't need either from a nutritional standpoint. Concentrating on vegetables is preferable and healthier.

The emphasis on dairy foods is a product of the National Dairy Council's biased promotion of dairy to nutrition programs at schools up to the university level.[44] In fact, there is some suggestion and concern that dairy is over-consumed in the Western diet.

Do not give your baby raw carrots, popcorn, peanuts, grapes, or other similarly hard to chew foods. I don't recommend popcorn or peanuts until the child is four years old or older. An infant can choke to death on a grape, or inhale a tiny bit of food into the lungs and end up with pneumonia. The hot dog remains the most common cause of choking death.[45]

I've heard of letting a baby teethe on a cold carrot, but the carrot won't dissolve in the throat if the infant is choking on it. A piece of zwieback or unsalted rice cake is preferable for teething foods. Teething rings are of little value and sales are aimed mostly to keep anxious parents occupied.

Some parents let infants eat crackers as finger foods. This is fine as long as you check the contents for salt, saturated fat, and sugar. Graham crackers are high in sugar or honey. It sticks to the older child's teeth and contributes to early cavities.

Now is the time to make your house safe. Not only do you need safety locks but you need to convert your house into a Nutritionally Safe Home. Control what foods are in the home. Yes, I know, your husband wants all that junk food and ice cream in the freezer! And, yes, you have another child who is skinny. This is the first step toward preventing your child from an addiction to fat, salt, and sugar. If you are serious about providing optimal nutrition to you child, then it is time to consider changing your home into a less toxic environment. Before you know it, your child will be entering school and this advice will no longer be practical. It is much easier to prevent habits than to break them.

In a safe house, limit or avoid totally: pickles, canned fruit, macaroni and cheese, Goldfish, doughnuts, "fresh squeezed organic juices" (they contain more sugar than Coke), and sugary cereals masquerading as food. Remember, if it has a Nutrition Facts label, it most likely is processed. Buy real foods, vegetables, fruit, and don't forget fish, lean meats, poultry, milk, and eggs.

Many commercial crackers contain 40% of their calories from fat and are loaded with salt. Although I'm not worried about the fat content during infancy, this is when habits begin. It has been demonstrated that a low salt diet in infancy protects against the development of high blood pressure later in life. Studies as early as 1997 shows that high blood pressure (hypertension) later in life may well be the price we pay for too much salt in childhood.[46]

FOOD NOTES ON LIQUIDS OTHER THAN MILK

It's nutritionally more sound to give the baby water than juice. If you choose to give juice, be certain that it is pasteurized, if not fresh, and limit it to only once a week. If your baby totes a bottle around all day for security, do not put diluted juice in it. Use pure water. Tap water is fine. If your water is not fluoridated and you don't use a fluoride supplement, bottled fluoridated water is a good option. It is healthier and won't destroy the infant's teeth or appetite for healthier foods.

I've seen many two year olds whose teeth were nearly rotted away from the ever-present bottle of diluted apple juice. And premature loss of primary teeth can lead to damage to the permanent teeth.[47] Because milk sugar, lactose, promotes cavities, rotting teeth are seen in nursing babies over a year of age when the mother uses her breasts as a pacifier.

Orange and other citrus juices can cause a contact rash around the mouth. The fresher the juice, the more peel oil is present in the juice. It is the peel oils that cause the irritation to the skin around the mouth, not citric acid. This is not allergy. Tomato sauce also contains a lot of peel oil, and also may cause skin irritation. If you wash the infant's face immediately after feeding foods with high peel oil content, these rashes may be avoided or decreased. Peel oil concentrations are controlled in the commercial production of all juices. Today's formulas are fortified with Vitamin C, and many non-citrus juices are too. Breast milk contains sufficient Vitamin C to protect your infant from scurvy.

Although 70% of parents with infants 6 months and under say they give juice to their babies, there is no nutritional need for it. Many juices have as much as 6 teaspoons of sugar in a small container. Fruit juice lacks the protein, fat, calcium, Vitamin D, iron, and zinc needed to support normal development in infancy and childhood. The Vitamin C in fruit itself is a more nutritious source than juice, and mother's milk has plenty of Vitamin C as well. Infant formulas are fortified with Vitamin C. How often have you seen scurvy?

This is but another baby food industry scam. They often use, "may enhance the immune system," to suggest the Vitamin C in juice will protect against the "common cold."

I don't understand why, but I find many nurses buying this untruth. Often I hear an RN saying, "I always take a high dose of Vitamin C as soon as I feel that I might be getting a cold." How I wish that really worked![48]

In the early 1970's, I had an epidemic of yellow-orange babies in my practice. It wasn't jaundice—the whites of their eyes were clear and the babies were vigorous—it was too much beta-carotene from carrot juice. Once they drank less carrot juice, the color disappeared. Carotene is also found in squash, sweet potato, and tomato. The color does not harm the baby. The real problem with carrot juice is that an important nutrient, fiber, is discarded during processing. Health conscious parents often try to avoid processed foods, and inadvertently do the processing themselves. There are now juicers available that retain the fiber and those are the preferred types. Fiber slows the absorption of the carrot sugars, but some nutritionists claim that blenders defeat the delaying effect of fiber. That is why I recommend smoothies to be avoided or served only once a week at most.

Prune juice is well tolerated by most infants and toddlers and is high in iron, but I haven't found it to be especially effective for constipation. Prunes or plums seem to have better results as natural laxatives for infants and children. If you prepare your own, look for prunes (at most health food stores) that don't contain sulfites as a preservative. If your child needs a natural laxative, figs, brown rice, spinach, and peas are excellent additional helpers.

Cola drinks, regular and diet soda, Kool Aid, Hi-C, Gatorade, sports and energy drinks, or punch have no place in an infant's diet. Or for that matter, in older children or teens. Carbonated beverages do not "settle" an upset stomach, and Gatorade is not good for an infant with diarrhea or dehydration. Sodas contain lots of sugar and in addition, phosphate, a compound that promotes calcium loss. This is hardly a time in an infant's development for that to happen.

Don't feed non-pasteurized eggnog or raw egg, honey, and banana blended as a milk shake—an "old wives" solution for putting weight on infants. Raw eggs often contain the salmonella germ and may also be very allergenic. Raw egg poses far more danger to the infant than low weight.

It's fine to give traditional breakfast foods for dinner and the vegetables, meat, and potatoes for breakfast. Most arrangements are cultural. Many Asian babies eat fish and rice for breakfast. The main meal in South and Central America is lunch. Furthermore, foods can be given more than once a day. In fact, many infants go on jags—preferring a particular food for days or weeks, then suddenly rejecting the food entirely and demanding something they wouldn't touch the week before. Don't let such temperamental tastes discourage you from reintroducing a rejected food on another day.

Commercially prepared baby foods are now being promoted as first step and second step foods. This is a marketing tactic. The latter are often referred to as junior foods. The difference between these foods is texture, not nutritional value. In fact, sugar is often added to these baby foods, so check the ingredients before purchasing them. They are designed to help the infant achieve a smooth transition to table foods. Generally second step foods are started at about 7 to 8 months of age; however, the age at which infants accept the more coarse texture is highly variable. Some children resist these lumpy foods until the end of the first year or even later. Do not feel that you must switch from strained foods.

You and your infant will decide how much of each food is appropriate. Don't force a baby to finish the jar or an arbitrary portion you've prepared. As a new father, I remember the games I made up to get that last teaspoon of food into my daughter's mouth. "Here comes the airplane into the hanger!" And just as I was congratulating myself on my slick maneuver, she'd gag and throw up the entire meal!

CHAPTER 10

Feeding Your Toddler and Preschooler

WHAT IS FAST FOOD?

Fast food is a food high in calories, sugar, fat, salt, and often caffeine. It is highly processed, "energy dense," and designed to be highly tasty. Many of the nutrients and fiber have been removed during processing. Lots of sugar and salt are added to improve flavor. In addition, these foods are conveniently packaged and highly advertised to children and parents over TV hundred of times a day. They invite busy parents to buy these foods for their children's lunch box. Pre-schools and hospitals unwittingly promote these foods from their vending machines. If you wish to see how fast foods have invaded our healthcare system, go to any hospital children's ward and take a look in their refrigerator! Thus a pattern is set early in life and often leads to addiction to junk food. Food preferences are formed before kids ever go to school. They get hooked on sugar at an early age and it becomes difficult to kick the habit with age. Prevention is easier than treatment of fast food/junk food addiction.

TODDLERS' TABLE FOODS

Most children begin to eat table foods between one and two years, which gives you one or two years from the baby's birth to clean up your nutritional act. Because even though you think you won't feed your toddler the kind of junk food you indulge in, she's almost certain to have other ideas. Babies especially desire the foods they see their parent eating. In no time at all, your valiant efforts—the careful nursing, homemade baby foods, conscientious avoidance of salt and extra sugars, reading all those labels—can come to nothing when your baby gets into your bag of potato chips or Goldfish.

Not only must you watch what you eat, you must watch what you don't eat. If you turn up your nose at broccoli or fish, your child is likely to do the same. Interestingly, for some reason children seem to emulate their fathers' food habits in particular. So fathers beware: you're the role model![49]

Babies at the toddler stage love finger foods. Get ready for spilled food, cereal mushed in the baby's hair and slathered all over his face, clothes, and your furniture. It's one big sticky mess for the next year or two!

Save the carpet by putting a plastic sheet under the high chair, or enlist a pet dog. But save your energy trying to teach table manners until the baby has developed better fine-motor coordination at about two-and-a-half to three years of age. When eating dissolves into playing, consider ending the meal promptly and allowing the child to leave the table.

Some toddlers are not yet ready for exclusive self-feeding. These children need help if they do not eat enough alone. There are children at this age who won't eat at all unless they are fed. Don't become upset, children vary in their readiness. In addition, some children are slow or pokey eaters. When they are rushed, they may leave the table before they're full, and go away hungry. I see this behavior often in kindergarten children who eat slowly. They feel they're missing all the fun playing outside with the children who wolfed down their lunch in a few moments. If your preschooler has this problem, discuss it with the teacher, who should allow your child more time to eat.

Toddlers who wait too long for meals often lose their appetites altogether, so don't hold a hungry child off until the rest of the family is ready to eat. Since most children thrive on regularity, try to serve your toddler his or her meals and snacks at roughly the same time each day. Nutritional snacking, or better-timed meals may be the answer.

Consistency, color, and texture of foods become increasingly important to the toddler, but just as important is not giving up feeding a particular food after a rejection. Some babies adapt slowly to new situations throughout life, and children with this inborn temperament often reject anything new, including new foods. This behavior fortunately can be modified once you understand that you have such a child. Keep reintroducing these rejected foods daily for about 20 days in a row. As familiarity develops, more often than not, your child will accept the food. The single biggest error a parent makes in food introduction is giving up after a few tries. On the other hand, it is important not to force the baby to eat a particular food. Just keep presenting the food daily until it is accepted.

Keep feeding time happy and relaxed. Good nutrition can easily break down at this point if the parent gives up and offers the child a special diet of crackers, grapes, raisins, peanut butter, and juice. A parent may believe that this diet is "better than nothing." What follows is a fight of wills, and the "persistent child" rules! Instead, keep eating time a happy time. If your child is not interested in the nutritious foods you prepare, allow him to leave the table to play. Save his dish of uneaten food for the time when he might be hungrier, but don't give him any other food. There are a few other "don'ts" as well. Don't bargain with your child or promise "a dessert" after he finishes his plate. Many studies have confirmed that this method often makes things worse. The slow-to-adapt, persistent child subsequently remembers the treat and a negative pattern of behavior quickly develops. Remember that the baby is rejecting the food and not your love. This confusion can easily creep into your feelings and cause frustration and anger. Your child may have the persistence, but not the judgment to make adult decisions. *Never forget who the adult is!* If you judge that a particular food is not good for your child, don't offer it as a bribe or reward and certainly not as standard fare.

Don't forget the effect of stress on your child's appetite. Stress of all kinds may have an effect on appetite: parental pressure to eat, divorce, separation, illness within the family, job loss, a new baby, new child care arrangement, a new school, a new home, or even an overly ambitious schedule can interfere with a child's appetite. Of course when a child is ill, one of the first things that happens is a decreased appetite. Unless it is a chronic illness, the appetite usually returns in about a week.

Soups with peas, carrots, small pieces of meat or chicken, brown rice, potato or noodles. Children who get introduced to soups at 8-9 months of age continue to like it when textures change from smooth to lumpy (but avoid those high sodium canned soups). Some babies gag on lumpy food until they are older and this is normal. Don't be in a hurry to advance textures too early. Avoid putting high salt food into the soup such as ham or sausage. The child will not miss it, but if the baby already is used to salt, the soup might be rejected at first. As stated above, don't give up. Remember the twenty times rule! Appear indifferent to any rejections and don't make a fuss over rejected foods. It usually makes things worse.

I suggest that you avoid serving Ramen noodles. They are extremely unhealthy because they are made by frying the noodles in saturated fat before drying. Top Ramen along with most instant cup of soups should be avoided at any age. Their high sodium and fat content make these easy to prepare items a poor choice for snack or lunch. Because they are inexpensive and easy to prepare they are a favorite food eaten by college kids. It remains on my "worst foods" list. The only thing missing in it is "radioactivity"!

Here are a few other suggestions for easy to prepare, nutritious finger foods, that make excellent snacks:

- Soft sweet peas
- Soft cooked carrot cubes
- Small pieces of very ripe banana
- Firm pieces of egg white or scrambled eggs
- Brown rice or small pieces of boiled potato (no French fries)
- Small pieces of poached/baked salmon, or white fish, such as tilapia
- Small pieces of boiled or baked chicken (skin removed)

MORE ON PICKY EATERS

Parents love "good eaters." They give back so much pleasure and that wonderful feeling of successful parenting. Mothers dream of the baby whose mouth is always ready for another morsel of "love." Then there is the nightmare baby who resists all initial attempts at being fed. These children can often be identified shortly after birth. As described above, they quickly undermine the confidence of the most secure parent!

My daughter called me recently, concerned that her two-year-old was too skinny. She asked if there were some vitamin, mineral supplement, or magic tonic that would boost his appetite. She was sure I would know what it was. Fortunately, I had kept her health records from the time she was a baby, and I faxed her the pertinent information. My daughter's height-weight proportions were almost exactly the same as her daughter at the same age. She was doing just fine. Inappropriate expectations can cause much anxiety in a parent. Remember that genetic factors and matters of temperament will also have something to do with how robust an eater your child will become.

Eating disorders often begin with the too-skinny two-year-old child whose parents make food the center of his existence. If your child refuses to eat as much as usual for more than a few days, don't be alarmed. This is often normal. The most common cause of a decrease in appetite is illness or a cold. Once the cold is over the appetite returns. Consult with your doctor if your child's appetite remains poor. But if your toddler looks well proportioned in spite of his "poor appetite," perhaps your expectations of how much food he needs is in error.

Several years ago, a foster parent called me because she believed her two and a half year old had emotional problems. She thought the cause might be the family's forthcoming move to a new community. The child was no doubt insecure, she said, though he need not be. The problem was his stealing food—from their plates at mealtime, and by slipping out of bed to raid the refrigerator in the middle of the night. The child was bloated from overeating, the foster mother told me, even though she had cut back on his regular meals in order to compensate for the extra food he was sneaking.

Your guess is correct. The little boy was starving. By the time I saw him, he was emaciated.

Although this is an extreme case, it demonstrates how errors in nutritional assessment can be made—even by educated, well-meaning people. These foster parents were both college graduates; the father was a minister. I'm convinced that neither of them would have purposefully done harm to the child they were raising. But our perceptions are clouded by personal bias as well as inexperience. For this reason, it's important to check in with your child's physician periodically to ensure that the child's weight and development are within normal ranges.

Well-child checks are designed to spot early problems and provide guidance—both important facets of preventive healthcare. It's a myth that left to their own choices, children will naturally select the food they need over a period of time. Most children in our culture gravitate toward the worst junk foods and some of the most potentially harmful non-nutritious snacks.

We can't really expect our kids, especially the very young ones, to resist fast food advertising propaganda, peer pressure, and vending machines. We haven't resisted.

But we must. Now's the time to get our nutritional house in order, even in the face of the most convincing pleas. Trust me. As the father of five, I've heard some pretty compelling reasons for buying Sugar Frosted Flakes, potato chips, and beef jerky.

As stated earlier, don't use food as a reward, and don't withhold food as a punishment. Give a toy, watch a video together, or take a trip to the zoo as recognition for your child's achievement for having put away his toys, for doing well in school. Avoid making "treat" synonymous with food or sweets.

How to Gently Break the Bottle and Pacifier Habit

Many parenting books recommend that a child's bottle be removed at one year to prevent tooth decay. A child may tote a bottle filled with juice (which is essentially sugar water) or milk all day and night. For those parents who feel the baby "needs" the bottle, it would be wise for them to put only water (never diluted juice) in the bottle and all "good" things, such as milk, go into a cup. This will make it easier for you to remove the bottle in the future when you feel you can handle the change. Here is one method of change to a cup that I have employed successfully over many years. It is virtually painless for the child and parent.

When the child is between fifteen to eighteen months old, put only water in the bottle as described above. After a week or two, tell your child that the "Bottle Man" is coming on Saturday to get all the bottles and pacifiers to give to the little babies. Even if you think the baby will not understand what you are saying, it is important that you repeat this message with a happy and enthusiastic voice. Saturday morning, before breakfast, collect all the bottles, nipples, caps, and pacifiers with your child and have him put them in a large paper shopping bag. Together, place the bag contents outside your front door and remind him in a happy and enthusiastic voice that the Bottle Man will be there to get these items for the little babies. Next, eat breakfast together. After breakfast remind your child about the bag and investigate to see whether the Bottle Man came. The bag should be empty of the bottles, but inside he should find a new teddy bear, or similar stuffed animal. Toy cars, trucks, or other items do not work as well as a stuffed animal. Explain that this is a present from the Bottle Man. Now the child can substitute this stuffed animal for the bottle as a security item and also cuddle it at bedtime. Instead of giving him a bottle at bedtime, cuddle your child in your lap and continue your bedtime ritual using a cup. Once you make the conversion, it is extremely important not to return to the bottle. If he asks for the bottle or pacifier, remind him that the Bottle Man gave them to the little babies, and give him the stuffed doll that the Bottle Man left for him or her! Do not attempt the conversion when your child is ill. Using this method, weekends are an ideal time to convert to a cup. The most common comment I get from parents is, "Had I known it would be so easy, I'd have done it sooner!"

Keep mealtimes pleasant and relaxed. Traditionally, the family gathers together at mealtime. In our culture we usually meet at the end of the day. This is a time to share our day's experience and what was nice about the day. This may not be the best time to discuss the disaster at school or frustration at work. Work on accentuating the positive when food is served. (And turn off the TV during mealtimes or cherished personal computer-phone!)

You will be getting much advice on what type of milk to give to your child. A fuss is being made over giving whole milk to your child or waiting to introduce low fat milk until he or she is over two years old. The truth of the matter is that 2% milk contains adequate fat for optimal brain growth and is the preferred type of milk for children between one and two. When children eat whole grains, vegetables, and meat too, they get a more than sufficient amount of fat for optimal growth and nutrition. One percent low fat milk is probably also fine for most children as well, but I usually reserve this for older children. I'm not aware of a single case of nutritional problems due to "too little fat" in children over a year old whose family followed this advice. If you have a child who is exceptionally thin, it is important that you consult your pediatrician or healthcare provider to re-evaluate your child's diet and health. A complete history and physical examination is needed. Don't attempt to "fatten the child up" with high saturated fat and sugary foods.[50]

CHAPTER 12

Snacks

When my son was born, he quickly adapted to an every-two-hours eating schedule. My wife kept asking me when this demanding schedule would change. Twenty-five years later she notes that it never has changed: he has breakfast, a mid-morning snack, lunch, an afternoon snack, dinner, and a snack before bed. His "grazing" six or more meals a day did not make him overweight. Calories do count, but his total calorie intake over 24 hours was sufficient to cover what he burned from activity plus his growth needs.

Eating between meals gets bad press, but I think this is more about what we eat than when we eat. The human digestive tract is especially well adapted to snack-type eating rather than three major meals a day. As long as what we're eating is low in percentage of calories from fat, sugar, low in salt and not totally without fiber as a result of consuming ultra refined snacks, nibbling throughout the day is no problem.

The problem is that many nibble-type foods are high in saturated fat, sugar, high in salt, and low in fiber. Potato chips, corn chips (even "health food store" chips), granola bars, trail mix, crackers, cookies, doughnuts, cupcakes, ice cream, soda, Kool Aid, Hi-C, juice, milkshakes, salted nuts, and a variety of candy bars, are examples. Remember, a low fat candy bar means a high sugar candy bar! Health food stores, drugstores, and supermarkets line their shelves with power bars, energy bars, and snack bars that are essentially candy bars, marketed with unsubstantiated claims that these candy bars are healthy snacks made with an "ideal ratio" of simple to complex carbohydrates, along with protein and fat. There is no proof that such an ideal ratio exists! The "staying power" of the "instant energy" sports or chocolate bars are platitudes invented by copy-writers.

Snacking is fine. Don't change the habit, change the choice of your snacks.

Children like simple snacks. Frozen bananas are a favorite treat for the two-year-old and older. Peel any overripe bananas, those with dark skins that you usually discard. Cut them in half, then place each half in a plastic Zip-Lock bag and freeze. Once frozen, simply serve—no preparation is required.

Whole wheat bagel and non-fat or 1% cream cheese is another favorite. Life is a compromise. There are many snacks that are not "perfect." Deviating from what is "ideal" on occasion should not be a big deal!

Don't forget cut-up fresh fruit, corn kernels (no added sugar), peas, or garbanzo beans. Hummus is made by blending chick peas (garbanzos), adding a few drops of lemon, and blending in favorite non-salt spices that your child likes. This is a more nutritious substitute for peanut butter or cream cheese. There are many excellent commercially prepared brands of hummus available at most grocery stores and Farmer's markets.

Another favorite is low-fat, low-salt vegetarian chili beans, prepared from scratch or from a can. Health Valley makes delicious, wholesome chili. Check their Nutrition Facts label.

Matzo and water crackers are better choices when coupled with low sodium mozzarella string cheese.

A whole wheat English muffin with low-salt tomato sauce and a slice of mozzarella cheese, microwaved, makes an instant pizza snack.

Small cut-up pieces of chicken breast, or for the older child, a baked chicken leg, sprinkled with paprika and served over a bowl of brown rice make an excellent school lunch, transported in a Tupperware-like container.

Air popped popcorn is an excellent choice for children over five years old. Younger children should avoid popcorn because it is easy to choke on.

Smoothies, especially on warm days, made with low or non-fat milk and seasonal fruit are nutritious and loved by most children, but no added sugar.

A forgotten snack food is the **chestnut**. Chestnuts are high in complex carbohydrates and contain a mere trace of fat. Two large chestnuts have less than 30 calories.

I have fond memories of street vendors roasting chestnuts over charcoal fires on cold winter afternoon and evenings. This was in Innsbruck, Austria, in the 1950's where I attended the University of Innsbruck when

I wasn't skiing! The smell of roasted chestnuts sold them. I bought them in small bags, and the process of peeling away the shell and inner skin warmed my frozen fingers.

Chestnuts are also good boiled and served with brussels sprouts or mashed and seasoned alongside small portions of lean roast meats. Introduce your family to chestnuts. It's a great snack food.

IDEAS FOR SNACKS AND LUNCHES AT HOME OR AFTER SCHOOL

These are suggestions when you run out of ideas

1. Grilled cheese sandwich using reduced fat sliced Swiss or Jack cheese on toasted whole grain bread. Use a non-stick skillet or microwave to melt the cheese. Low-fat and reduced fat cheese taste better if it is melted.

2. Exra lean ground beef, brown rice, and ketchup mixed and fried together in a skillet, then packed in a Tupperware-like container for transportation. Quinoa may be substituted for rice. Most kids love this!

3. Baked apple, plain or with yogurt.

4. Meatloaf sandwich.

5. Tuna salad sandwich made with 50% less salt tuna and mayonnaise or low-fat yogurt. Make with a whole wheat slice of bread on one side and white bread on the other side.

6. Fresh fruit salad.

7. Bowl of low-sodium chili, vegetarian or with very lean meat.

8. Chicken sandwich using low-salt ketchup as a spread, or mayonnaise. Corn on the cob. When not in season, a bowl of washed frozen corn kernels mixed with green peas (look for no added sugar brands). A zip-lock type bag makes this mixture transportable.

9. Boca Burger or Veggie Burger (vegetarian "hamburger" found in many health food stores frozen section) grilled, and served on a toasted bun with ketchup, slice of butter lettuce, and slice of ripe tomato. Use sliced cherry tomatoes when vine-ripened tomatoes are not available.

10. Extra-lean roast beef sandwich with favorite whole-grain roll. Use mustard or ketchup as a spread. Serve with a banana or slice of melon.

Have a side dish of small boiled potatoes, broccoli florets, and sliced steamed carrots.

11. Hamburger made with extra-lean ground beef. Add some rice or quinoa and low-sodium chicken broth to the meat mixture to keep it moist and enhance its flavor. For variety, try mixing in a little mustard or barbecue sauce. Add a crisp apple or ripe seasonal fruit.

12. Meatloaf sandwich. Raw carrots and cherry tomatoes. Mixed dehydrated fruit.

13. Cup of pea soup using one of the many low-sodium, low-fat brands. Baked skinless drumettes of chicken, sprinkled with sweet paprika over rice. Slice of cantaloupe or cubes in a bowl with blueberries when in season.

14. Boiled, steamed, or microwaved corn on the cob, without any salt, but a little "I Can't Believe It's Not Butter," if desired. Broiled skinless chicken breast, plain or sliced thin on a bun with fresh salsa as a topping. Fresh orange, peeled.

15. Small bowl of macaroni with grated low-fat cheese, such as Kraft shredded reduced-fat mozzarella, sprinkled over it and microwaved until the cheese melts. A fruit smoothie with milk and no added sugar.

16. Nachos and a bowl of low sodium beans. (Don't forget the Beano—2–3 drops with the first bite!) Strawberry-banana plus low fat milk smoothie.

17. Fresh toasted whole wheat bagel with hummus or low-fat whipped cream cheese. Raw celery and raw carrots. Edamame—cooked soy beans (pronounced "eh-dah-MAH-may") are fun to eat and easy to serve. Add a hard-boiled egg.

18. Bowl of medium sized shrimp and salsa. Baked potato with low-fat sour cream and chives. Use salsa as topping for potato as well, if desired. (Check the sodium content per serving on the food label.)

19. Leftover whole wheat/regular spaghetti or macaroni with low-sodium tomato meat sauce. Serve heated or cold. Transportable in a "Tupperware-like" container. Fresh apple. 1 or 2% milk. Avoid chocolate milk because it may contain 14 grams or more (about 3.5 teaspoons) of added sugar!

20. Turkey sandwich made with unprocessed, real turkey (avoid the highly-processed high-sodium turkey rolls). Use cranberry sauce as a spread. Mashed potato, baked yam, or sweet potato.

21. Pita bread (pocket bread) stuffed with shredded lettuce, cooked ground lean hamburger meat, or cooked ground turkey, and low-fat, low-sodium salad dressing on top.

22. Beef or turkey tacos with shredded lettuce, tomato, and shredded low-fat cheese. Glass of 1 or 2% milk. Whole wheat fig bars (buy a no-sugar added brand).

23. Cold, leftover broiled salmon sandwich served with low-sodium salad dressing as a spread, lettuce, and slice of ripe tomato. A salmon salad with medley of vegetables is another variation.

24. Omelet made with two egg whites and one yolk. Cubed vegetable sauté, shredded mozzarella cheese, and lean low-sodium ham, diced for the inside. Served with reduced sodium salsa over the top when cooked. Serve with a fresh whole wheat toasted bagel and very small boiled new potatoes.

25. Egg salad sandwich. Unsalted or low-sodium whole wheat pretzels.

26. Banana bread, cornbread, or potato latkes with apple sauce.

27. Sliced kiwi, dry cereal (Shredded Wheat, Kashi Heart to Heart) and 1 or 2% milk.

28. Turkey hamburger. Fresh orange slices.

29. Salmon sandwich on rye or whole wheat bread. (Canned salmon mixed with mayo and chopped scallions plus sliced cherry tomatoes with butter lettuce on top.)

30. Don't forget the ten super-foods: Sweet potatoes, whole grain bread, broccoli, organic strawberries, beans, cantaloupe, spinach, kale, oranges, oatmeal, and 1–2% fat milk.

POOR CHOICE SNACKS & BREAKFAST CEREAL

- Apple juice: Pure sugar water
- Cap'n Crunch: High sugar and very low fiber
- Capri-Sun: Sugar water
- Cheeseburger: Very high saturated fat and sodium
- Cheeze-It: Almost no fiber and too much sodium
- Chicken nuggets: High in saturated fat

- Cocoa Puffs: High sugar cereal with almost no fiber
- French fries: High fat and sodium with almost no fiber
- Froot Loops: High in sugar and little fiber
- Gatorade: Very high sugar, water is preferred for rehydration
- Goldfish: High fat, high sodium, and low in fiber
- Hormel SPAM: Extremely high in sodium
- Hot dogs: Very high in saturated fat and sodium
- KRAFT Macaroni and Cheese: Very high in saturated fat and sodium—An introduction to hypertension
- Lucky Charms: High in sugar and almost no fiber
- Lunchables: High saturated fat, sodium, and sugars
- Pickles: Extremely high in sodium, a significant promoter of hypertension
- Rice Krispies: Calories, air, and no fiber. Better used in a chocolate bar!
- V8: Very high in sodium—a high blood pressure cocktail
- Anything with alfredo sauce!

CHAPTER 13

Information about Real Foods

When we think of sugar, we generally imagine that white crystalline product—but that's just the tip of the sugar iceberg. Sugar exists in most foods we eat: juice, soda, jams, cookies, chocolate, crackers, hot and dry cereals, pies, ice cream, chili, pizza, Jell-O, hot dogs, bacon, ham, salami, cold cuts, stuffings, breads, soups, mayonnaise, catsup, salad dressing, fruit flavored yogurt, canned vegetables, beans, and virtually all frozen foods, to name just a few. The average American consumed approximately 120 lbs of sugar a year in 1998, which is a tremendous amount. It must be 50% more now in 2020!

Besides refined cane and beet sugar, chemically known as sucrose, products may contain refined fructose, glucose, dextrose, lactose, levulose, or maltose. All of these refined sugars have been stripped of their mineral, vitamin, and fiber content. They are good as a sweetener and for calories; whereas nutritious foods such as oranges, blackberries, blueberries, strawberries, cantaloupe, apples, plums, papaya, mango, and dried fruits are all high in sugar but retain the important vitamins, minerals, and fiber. The sugar in these foods is absorbed more slowly by the body compared with refined sugars or juices. Other refined sugars such as corn syrup, molasses, maple syrup, and honey are absorbed rapidly and stress the hormones in our body that maintain balance or homeostasis. "Sugarless" desserts and ice cream are sometimes deceptively loaded with honey or "real maple syrup." Although many parents or children may prefer a particular type of sugar, the body uses all sugars in essentially the same way. None of these sugars are nutritionally better than cane sugars, and brown sugar, raw sugar, honey, or molasses are not any healthier than other sugars.

Finally the Nutrition Facts label found on all packaged foods and beverages must now state the amount of *sugar added* to a food or drink. This is an important advance, thanks to public pressure groups such as the Center for Science in the Public Interest.

Apple juice is probably the greatest source of sugar in a small child's diet. It should be limited to a single 6 oz. bottle or cup a week (at the most), and not toted around in the bottle. "Watered-down" juice is very popular, but is especially damaging to the teeth and appetite when consumed throughout the day (and night). Baby food companies cunningly promote juice by strategically placing rows of juice bottles above the desirable baby fruit and vegetable jars! An infant has no nutritional need for juice. Formula and breast milk provide an infant with enough water even in hot weather. Breast milk also contains lots of sugar (lactose or milk sugar). Infants who breastfeed past a year of age, especially as a calming agent, all day and throughout the night, often develop severely decayed teeth. This habit can lead to diseased permanent teeth.

The impact on behavior from eating sugar and various foods has been a topic of both interest and concern to parents. There is now considerable evidence that the concern about sugar consumption as presented by the media is understated. However, the myths surrounding sugar, including the myth of the "sugar high" or that it causes hyperactivity, have been slow to disappear.[51] These myths are misleading and harmful. We need to place sugar in the diet in perspective. Small amounts of sugar have an important place in nutrition. For example, the only fuel the brain uses is sugar. Actually there is some evidence showing sugar to have a calming effect on normal and hyperactive children. Too much sugar, on the other hand, like too much of anything, is detrimental to our health and eating too much sugar does contribute to tooth decay, obesity, constipation, malnutrition, heart disease, type 2 diabetes, and the metabolic syndrome. A major issue is that there is no RDA (Recommended Dietary Allowance) for sugar. So when one says, "a little bit," what does that mean?

Fructose and high fructose corn syrup (HFCS) are in the headlines now and for good reason. Fructose may be the driver of metabolic syndrome. Sucrose breaks down into glucose and our enemy fructose. Are these sugars toxic? Are they addictive? The evidence is mounting and sugar is ubiquitous. Even Gerber and Heinz add sugars to more than half of their Second Stage and Third Stage fruit and some vegetables. Sport juices and fruit juices, berry juices along with sodas line the supermarket and grocery store shelves. Are these poisons? I don't know, but my recommendation is to keep these drinks out of your home and out of your food except for special holidays and occasions.

We are now in the midst of an obesity epidemic. Much of it is a result of consuming high-sugar drinks, overeating, and lack of exercise. Many of my obese and overweight patients confess to drinking 6–8 large sodas, sugar drinks, or juices a day. That's well over 50 teaspoons of sugar a day and that does not include the sugar from their ice cream, candy bars, energy bars, and multiple other sources. When I go to the movies I see the long lines leading up to the "food" concession where super-sized drinks, ice cream, hot dogs, pizza, chips, nachos, and giant-sized candy bars are sold. Once in the theater, the screen reminds us there is still time to get some more. Don't starve or become dehydrated during a tense two-hour movie!

As they say, "A second in your mouth, a minute in the stomach, and the rest of your life (as fat) on your hips, butt, and gut!" Think of that before taking your first bite. Let's face it, who can eat only one or two potato chips and then put the bag away? Better to resist the first bite. If you are not able to follow this advice, seek out a 12-step program

EGGS

Unless your child or you have eczema or has already shown an allergy to eggs, this food may safely be introduced to a child over age one, or earlier in many cultures.

The egg is composed of egg white, one of the purest and best proteins available, and the egg yolk, a repository for cholesterol and protein. Interestingly, people with already high LDL cholesterol levels (over 100mg) don't experience much of an increase in their blood cholesterol level by eating eggs, whereas people with normal LDL cholesterol (less than 100mg) show a dramatic increase in cholesterol when they eat eggs.[52]

Infants may need diets higher in cholesterol and fats than adults, but this should not be interpreted to mean that you must go out of your way to introduce high saturated fat or high cholesterol foods.

Egg yolk had traditionally been introduced to children early because it had the reputation of being a great source of iron. But now we know that the iron in egg yolk is poorly absorbed by the body. I'm especially wary of large amounts of egg yolk because environmental poisons such as pesticide residues, which contaminate animal feeds, may show up in concentrated amounts in animal organs such as liver, eggs, and chicken skin.

On the other hand, egg white is an excellent non-fat uncontaminated source of protein. Boil an egg. Pop out the yolk and discard it if environmental residues are a concern. Chop up the white to garnish the salads of the older child. One to three eggs a week for a young child are nutritionally wholesome as long as they are not fried or prepared with butter, lard or bacon fat.

FERTILE AND UNGRADED EGGS

A belief in "vitalism" prompts some people to buy fertilized eggs. From a nutritional point of view, fertilized and unfertilized eggs are identical. The more important issue is that raw fertile eggs are a dangerous threat to health. Graded eggs are sanitized using an antiseptic wash. Fecal germs on egg shells that haven't been through the antiseptic process cause hundreds of cases of food poisoning a year in the United States. Symptoms of salmonella food poisoning, which include nausea, vomiting, diarrhea, abdominal cramps, chills, fever, and achy muscles, usually begin 12–24 hours after eating contaminated food. Children, the elderly, and anyone with a compromised immune system are especially vulnerable to food poisoning.

Cartons of eggs sold in most supermarkets generally meet USDA Grade A requirements. To be certain, never eat raw or uncooked eggs. Even graded eggs are often contaminated. It is dangerous to put any raw egg in a "milkshake." Unpasteurized eggnog or Caesar salad dressing are extremely risky and should be avoided.

TOFU

Tofu is a non-meat, non-dairy source of protein that is relatively high in calcium and low in price. It has been an important part of the Asian diet for more than 2,000 years. Today, most supermarkets and health food stores carry it. It's prepared from soybeans that have been soaked overnight, ground, boiled, strained, made into curd, cut into blocks, and kept refrigerated. Three-and-a-half ounces, or about 1/2 cup, contain about 145 calories and 8–10 grams of protein. Furthermore, soybean is a complete protein, that is, it contains all the essential amino acids. Although 3.5 oz of tofu contain 9 grams of fat, it is cholesterol free and the fat is mostly polyunsaturated.

Tofu can be added to soup and salads, or barbecued. It can be stir-fried, broiled, grilled, sautéed, or baked. It can be pureed to make dips, spreads, salad dressing, and, when mashed, it can be substituted for ricotta or cottage cheese.

There are two basic types of tofu, soft and firm. Soft tofu comes in thick, straight-edged blocks; the firm type has compressed edges. When you buy tofu, check the date for freshness. Rinse the tofu when you get it home, place it in a container of fresh cold water, and store it in the refrigerator. Change the water daily.

Miso is another soy product. It is a salty seasoning paste made from a combination of soybeans and a grain such as rice or barley. This product should be avoided because its sodium content can exceed 900 milligrams per tablespoon (see my discussion on salt or sodium).

POTATO

Along with rice, corn, and wheat, the potato is known worldwide as a staff of life. Spanish conquistadors carried it to Europe from the Andes in the 16th century, and it has become one of the most nutritious and versatile food staples.

It's a wonderful food: a medium-size potato contains only 100 calories, is 99.9% fat free, and provides about half the Vitamin C a person needs in a day. Potato skin is high in dietary fiber and contains most of the Vitamin C. Although the potato isn't particularly rich in protein, its biological quality is as high or higher than the soybean protein. The downside to potato may be that it rapidly turns to sugar when eaten or digested.

People associate the Irish with potatoes, but I think of eastern Europe. My mother prepared potato soup, boiled potatoes, baked potatoes, and mashed potatoes. Remembering her potato latkes, potato kugel, and potato knaedel still makes my mouth water. By the time of her death at age 94, she had supplied me with a generous variety of traditional Jewish potato recipes that I still cherish. Sadly, Americans have veered away from the wholesome use of potatoes. More than half of the potatoes we eat these days are in the form of potato chips, processed frozen French fries, fast-food French fries, and dehydrated potato preparations. In 1980, Americans ate five billion pounds of French fries, and one billion pounds of potato chips. While an 8-ounce potato has 140 calories, 8 ounces of potato chips contain 1200 calories, 28 teaspoons-full (133 grams) of which are pure fat! And that does not even include the salt load.

While you still have some say in the matter, avoid starting your toddler on these foods. Stick to something wholesome such as basic mashed potatoes. But once again, beware! Potato rapidly breaks down in the body to sugar, and for the anti-sugar advocates, this food is on their list of "forbidden fruit."

RICE

Rice is one of the most nutritious grains. It is the principal food for many millions of people throughout the world. Most children quickly learn to love rice. Although it doesn't contain an unusually high percentage of protein, it is of higher biological value than corn. One half cup of rice contains about three grams of protein. Unpolished rice, such as brown rice, contains bran, a dietary fiber, in its husk. The husk is now being studied to see if it contains any anti-diabetes factors. Rice bran lowers blood cholesterol as much as oat bran, but unlike oat bran, rice bran doesn't turn gummy when cooked. You can buy rice bran which is packaged like wheat germ and is used in similar ways. Sprinkle it on cereal, salad, and low-fat yogurt, or add it to baked goods. An ounce contains 8 grams of dietary fiber, 4 grams of protein, and lots of niacin, thiamin, magnesium, and iron.

In the 1890's there was a strange outbreak of an illness called beriberi in Asia characterized by fatigue, weight loss, emotional disturbances, impaired sensory perception, weakness and pain in the limbs, swelling of the body tissues, staggering gait, heart failure, and death. Some of the best physicians in the world were sent to study it. Dr. Christiaan Eijkman, a Dutch physician, was sent to Indonesia to study this illness. He lived in a home to observe a family with these symptoms. This home had a yard with chickens and goats as did many homes at that time. The diet of the family was mostly polished rice. Polished rice was developed, not because of its taste, but because brown rice has a short shelf life, while polished rice has a very long shelf life. One day the family ran out of the regular chicken feed usually used. Instead, the family began feeding their left over white rice to the chickens. Soon Dr. Eijkman noticed that the chickens began to become very aggressive and developed poor balance, stumbling and soon dying, similar to the family's beriberi.[53]

Dr. Eijkman decided to feed the chickens unpolished brown rice. The chickens recovered! This was a "nutritional disease" and it was cured by consuming the unprocessed rice containing husks. The husk contained an anti-beriberi factor. This is how thiamine or Vitamin B-1 was discovered. Dr. Eijkman was awarded the Nobel Prize.

Most of this has been forgotten because white rice was "enriched" with vitamins and beriberi became almost an historical illness.

Now there is an epidemic of diabetes mellitus type2 in Asia, as there is in the USA. But the difference is that in India, Indonesia, the Philippines,

Vietnam, and China, the illness is not necessarily associated with obesity, as it is in the USA.

Recalling the beriberi epidemic, scientists once again began studying polished rice and found that those who consumed large amounts of rice 5 times a week were at high risk for developing diabetes mellitus type 2 while those who consumed brown rice had over 15% lower risk for developing it. Brown rice appears to be protective. If the white rice was replaced with whole grains, including brown rice, this was associated with a 35% lower diabetes risk. This data supports the recommendation that most carbohydrate intake should come from whole, unrefined grains. Many endocrinologists dismiss this and say it is all due to a high carbohydrate diet. Stay tuned![54]

FORMS OF RICE

Short and medium grain rice is wetter than long rice and their kernels stick together. You can overcome the stickiness by adding oil to the water in which you cook the rice, but by now you know I wouldn't recommend any type of oil. Don't add salt either. If you don't like sticky rice, use long grain or parboiled rice.

Long grain rice is generally preferred for Chinese cooking and is good for curries, pilaf, or stews served over rice. The stickier rice is especially good for puddings or molded rice dishes, California roll sushi, and many Japanese dishes.

Kernels that break during the milling process are sold as **"broken rice,"** which is a little less expensive than other rice.

Whole grain rice, as opposed to **polished rice,** retains all the grain's nutrients, most notably vitamins and minerals otherwise lost in milling when the outermost husk is removed. **Brown whole grain rice** is a popular favorite. It has a nice nut-like flavor and is chewier than white rice. Short grain brown rice is even chewier than the long grain version.

Polishing or processing rice, as stated earlier, involves removing the outer layer. Polished rice has been discredited because it is deficient in B Vitamins. Polished rice has a lower fat content than brown rice, so it is less likely to become rancid. The reason for the popularity of white rice is increased shelf life. Supposedly polished rice also creates less gas in the bowels because it has less bran than the whole grain.

Enriched rice is polished rice to which iron, thiamine, and niacin have been returned in amounts approximating those that of un-milled kernels. Uncle Ben's is a popular, easy to prepare "enriched" rice. You get the three B-Vitamins and iron that are added to all enriched grains, but you lose the fiber, magnesium, Vitamins E and B-6, copper, zinc, and other nutrients such as the poorly understood phytochemicals (plant chemicals) that are in the whole grains, like brown rice.

Parboiled or **converted white rice** has been specially treated to retain vitamins. It may contain two to four times as much thiamine and niacin as polished white rice. The term "parboiled" is slightly misleading as the rice is not precooked, but is actually somewhat harder than regular rice. It takes a little longer to cook than regular white rice, but the grains will be very fluffy and separate after they have been cooked. My personal favorites are long grain brown rice, the brown delicious rice found in many Thai restaurants.

Precooked rice has been fully cooked and dehydrated after milling. This is the "instant" or "minute rice" that needs no preparation beyond pouring boiling water over the rice according to the package directions, and letting stand for a few minutes before serving. This stuff is pretty tasteless and less nutritious than other rice. The newest addition to instant rice is precooked converted rice that has been vacuum-packed in a plastic bag. Simply immerse it in boiling water as directed on the package and in a few moments you have perfectly prepared rice.

Arborio is a starchy white rice with an almost round grain. This is the rice used to make the Italian dish risotto and it also works well for paella and rice pudding. Arborio absorbs up to five times its weight in liquid as it cooks, which results in grains of a creamy consistency.

Wild rice is botanically unrelated to rice. It is a grain native to North America. Like rice, it grows in marshy land. French explorers found it growing around the Great Lakes and called it "crazy oats," although it is no more related to oats than to rice. Because it is difficult to produce in large quantities, wild rice is extremely expensive. It has a distinct nutty flavor and chewiness. Yum Yum.

CORN, WHEAT, QUINOA, AND OTHER GRAINS

Technically a grass, corn is the only cereal born and bred in America. It was the main food of the Indian or indigenous civilizations of the Americas from the Canadian border to the Andes. The Pilgrims from England who settled here learned from the natives how to use corn.

The dried corn kernel is strong and hard on the outside, while its germ, or inside, is soft and almost floury. Indians showed the southern colonists how to pound, grind, and boil whole kernels in lye or lime water to make hominy, which remains a staple in the Southern diet. "Grits" refers to the flint-like, grainy, textured part of the kernel. (Unless cornmeal is soaked in water to soften it, the cornbread made from it is gritty.)

Toddlers tend to love corn bread, corn muffins, hominy grits, and corn flakes—all high in nutrients. Popcorn is one of the few popular snack foods that tastes good and provides solid food value, when not doused with butter, oil, or salt as served in the movie theaters. I don't recommend popcorn for children under five because of the possibility of choking.

My favorite form of corn is on the cob. A few years ago I planted eight rows of Eastern white corn in our big backyard garden, but because I planted them all together, we had five or six dozen ears of corn ready to be eaten all at the same time. Some farmer I turned out to be!

Our solution was a neighborhood "Pick Your Own" party and feast that was a huge success. It was the first time I had ever tried corn without butter or salt. It was fantastic!

If you buy fresh corn from a farmer's market, take along a cooler. Warm temperatures quickly convert the corn's sugar to starch. Select corn with plump, juicy, well-aligned kernels that are tightly packed. Buy those ears of corn with the husks still on, and discard ears with rusty looking tips or shriveled kernels.

To steam sweet corn, heat it through for about 2–5 minutes. To grill, cut off tassels, remove the silk, leave the husks on and soak in ice water for 5 minutes. Place over the coals, a few inches from the fire's center. Turn every 5 minutes. In 15 minutes, the husk should be blackened and the corn ready to eat.

WHEAT

The most widely grown of all cereal grains, wheat is a kind of berry that consists of an outer covering, the bran, which is high in minerals, B Vitamins, and some protein; and the inner part, or endosperm, which consists mainly of starch and protein. The wheat germ resides in the endosperm. The germ is comparatively high in fat and Vitamin E.

Wheat is made into white flour and whole wheat flour: White flour consists of ground endosperm only. Whole wheat or graham flour contains the bran and the entire endosperm. Because it contains the germ, which contains fat, whole wheat flour can spoil, whereas white flour can be stored fresh for much longer. On the other hand, whole wheat flour contains more fiber, minerals, vitamins, and slightly more protein than even enriched white flour (white flour to which thiamine, riboflavin, niacin, and iron have been added). Your toddler will enjoy whole wheat pasta, pilaf, and breads of many kinds if introduced early in life. Bulgur wheat, very high in fiber, is made from several varieties of wheat. It is used as a cereal, in soups or salads, as a side dish or main meal. Too much can cause gassiness.

If your children have grown used to white bread, help them switch to whole wheat by preparing sandwiches with one slice of white and one slice of whole wheat bread. Another way to introduce whole wheat bread is to switch to a bread that looks like whole wheat but has the texture of white, such as Roman Meal. This will let your child adapt to the color of whole wheat over a couple of weeks or even a month. Then switch to a mild whole wheat bread. The older the child, the slower the transition, especially with the slow to adapt, resistent child. Be patient and persistent —the long term gains are worth it.

RYE

Rye has a stronger, heartier flavor than wheat, and is typically used to make rye bread. Today's American rye bread is usually one-third rye flour, two-thirds whole wheat flour. When I was growing up it was the real thing, a traditional Jewish rye with caraway seeds and a crunchy crust. Onion and corn rye breads were my favorites. Authentic black pumpernickel, and German or Russian rye breads are also delicious, and you can find them in small local bakeries. They're worth hunting for.

Generally speaking, food from grains such as corn, wheat, or rye are among the most nutritious foods we eat as long as we don't add butter, "rendered chicken fat with onion" (my father's favorite), or margarine.

For the five-year-old, try low-fat cheese, lettuce, and ripe tomato sandwiches on rye. Many children do not develop a taste for lettuce until four years of age, so don't be too upset if your toddler rejects salads. Keep trying, and be sure to make a salad a daily part of the adult diet. Remember, you're the role model!

OATS

Oats are an ancient grain, probably cultivated since the first century AD. They are used most frequently as cattle food. Humans consume only about 5 % of the world oat crop. In America, oats are used mostly for hot cereal and more recently for muffins, cookies, and breads. Oats are an excellent source of complex carbohydrate and contain about 50% more protein than bulgur wheat, and twice as much as brown rice. They are rich in Vitamin E and the B Vitamin, folate, as well as the minerals iron, copper, zinc, and manganese. Oats are also a good source of dietary fiber, both soluble and insoluble. The soluble fiber is primarily responsible for lowering blood cholesterol. Two ounces of dry oats (1-1/3 cups cooked) contain 5 grams of fiber and only one gram of fat.

Granola is made from oats, but many commercial brands are extremely high in fat. Often highly saturated tropical oil, such as palm or coconut oil, is added to the oats before they are toasted. You can buy low fat granola or you can make your own. Toast quick or old-fashioned rolled oats on a baking sheet in a 300 F oven and stir frequently. If you wish, stir in honey to taste before toasting. Be careful not to scorch. After toasting, mix in your choice of wheat germ, bran, and chopped dried fruits. Let cool in a plastic bag or refrigerator.

Muesli is a cold cereal, very popular in Switzerland, Germany, and Austria. Like granola, mass-market muesli is often high in saturated fat and calories, but you can prepare your own fairly easily. Mix uncooked rolled oats with rolled wheat flakes, bite-sized shredded wheat, wheat nuggets, 100% bran shreds, oat or wheat bran, or wheat germ. Stir in any of your favorite dried fruits and a small amount of unsalted, coarsely chopped nuts or seeds. If you prefer sweet muesli, add a little brown sugar, maple syrup, or molasses. Serve only to children over three or four because younger children may choke on the seeds. Store in an airtight container in the refrigerator. If muesli is mixed with reduced fat milk and refrigerated overnight it will have the consistency of cooked cereal. If you prefer it crunchy, stir in reduced fat milk or low-fat yogurt just before serving.

ETHNIC GRAINS

Buckwheat isn't related to wheat, and isn't even a cereal. Technically or botanically, it's a fruit. In any case, it's another wonderful complex carbohydrate around which to build a meal. In middle European countries, buckwheat groats, or kernels, are prepared similarly to rice and called kasha. It is necessary to roast the kasha before boiling as roasting keeps it from developing a sticky, porridge-like consistency. Kasha and yogurt is an ethnic favorite among Eastern European Jews, as is "kasha varnishkas," kasha with bow-tie noodles. The kernels can also be processed into flour for pancakes or waffles.

Barley, sold whole or pearled (with the tough though nutritious bran covering removed), is another delicious complex carbohydrate that not many Americans know about. In this country, barley is used more as a source of malt for beer production, but, cooked with raisins and grated lemon peel, it makes a nutritious and delicious cereal high in fiber, iron and other nutrients. It's also good in casseroles and soups. Aside from the flavor, I love the chewy texture of this grain.

Millet is a term applied to a variety of small seeds used mainly for birdseed in this country, but in Africa, India, and China, millet is a staple grain. The most popular millets are sorghum, the premier cereal in Africa, used in the U.S. mostly for sorghum syrup; or pearl millet, which you can usually find in "health" food stores for use as a cereal, or in meal form. Millet is used to make porridge in North Africa and roti (a flat bread) in India.

Quinoa pronounced "keen-wah" is technically a seed, not a grain and is grown high in the Andes Mountains of South America. This pseudo-cereal is not a member of the true grass family. The nutrient composition is very good compared with common cereals. It is a good source of protein, fiber, calcium and is therefore an excellent food for vegans and those who are lactose intolerant or truly have celiac disease. Quinoa contains no gluten or wheat. It cooks very easily, in about 15 minutes. Cook it in a pot as you do rice. Cook it at a high setting until is starts boiling and then cover and simmer for about 12–15 minutes. Be careful not to use too much water otherwise it will take longer to cook. Stir the quinoa so all the water gets absorbed.

It can be used instead of pasta and served with marinara sauce over it.

BEANS, PEAS, LENTILS, AND OTHER LEGUMES

Legumes are vegetables that come in pods. They include all beans, often named for their shape or color: kidney, black, pink, red, or white; peas, which are usually round but also grow elongated and multicolored like black-eyed peas; and lentils, flat, disk-like legumes that are green or pink or orange and are sold whole or split. The peanut is also a legume, not a nut.

White beans, red beans, kidney beans, black-eyed peas, lentils, and garbanzos are all similar in content—they are outstanding complex carbohydrates, low in fats and salt, and high in fiber. They are also very economical, and among the most nourishing of vegetables. Use them in casseroles and soups, in salads, or as a side dish. They're also a good source of water-soluble vitamins, especially thiamine, riboflavin, niacin, and folate.

Red, white, and kidney beans, black-eyed peas, lentils, and garbanzos are generally packaged dried, and most are available canned or frozen. Dried peas and beans lose their nutritional value after about a year of storage. Frozen and canned beans usually contain too much salt, but canned no-salt added legumes are now showing up in most grocery stores.

Aside from highest grades for nutritional and economic value, beans are rich in anti-carcinogenic substances that may help prevent or control certain cancers. Soybeans contain a particular type of anti-carcinogen that may reduce the risk of some hormone-dependent cancers, such as breast or prostate.

"Beano" is sold in most grocery and health food stores as an aid to reduce gassiness. It is a digestive aid. When a couple of drops of this digestive enzyme is added to your first spoonful of beans or lentils, the result are like magic! It is usually very effective, practically tasteless, and safe. For those of you unable to tolerate legumes because of gassiness, I highly recommend this additive. It is also safe for toddlers. Follow the directions on the label.

TREE NUTS, PEANUTS, AND PEANUT BUTTER

Nuts and peanuts are an important part of the older child or adult diets, as long as not coated with sugar or salt. And once again I wish to remind you that the peanut is dangerous to younger children because it is easily aspirated into the lungs and cause severe lung damage.

Peanut butter is like putty and a large amount can easily block the back of a child's throat.

Peanuts contain aflatoxin, a naturally occurring carcinogen and liver toxin that is produced by mold on damp peanuts.[55] Roasting does not destroy this heavy-duty toxin. The US Department of Agriculture has a good program in place to minimize aflatoxin contamination of peanuts in commercially processed peanut butters and it seems to be keeping contamination down to acceptably low levels. But "real" peanut butter, made from ground peanuts in a home processor or at the health food store is believed to have ten times the amount of aflatoxin as the Skippy or Jif type brands.

Dentists warn against the peanut butter and jelly sandwich. It plasters jelly (sugar) against the teeth and if not removed quickly, may contribute to cavities.

OLDER CHILDREN LOVE NUTS AND SEEDS

Unsalted almonds and walnuts make nutritious snacks and should be a part of a prudent diet. They are high in protein and essential fatty acids. Almonds are a good source of omega-6 fats as found in vegetable oils. Walnuts on the other hand are rich in omega-3 fatty acids, the same type that comes from salmon and fatty fish. A 4-6 gram serving contain 95% of the daily value of omega-3 fatty acids. Unfortunately, too few children and teenagers eat nuts regularly. A small handful of almonds or walnuts can provide filling protein, fiber, unsaturated fats plus vitamins and minerals. They lower cholesterol levels and the anti-inflammatory power of omega-3 fatty acid may be cardio-protective.

Other unsalted nuts include hazelnuts, Brazil nuts, pecans, pistachios, and cashews. But beware! Nuts are also small bundles of calories! Avoid the salted versions.

For older children, don't forget seeds, such as unsalted sunflower and pumpkin seeds.

YELLOW VEGETABLES

Yellow vegetables are rich in beta carotenes, which convert to Vitamin A when eaten. Carrots, squash, yams, or sweet potatoes are examples of vegetables loaded with carotenes. Yellow corn and cantaloupe are also rich in Vitamin A or beta carotene. If you are looking for foods high in Vitamin A, think yellow.

Fortunately, most children love carrots. The younger child should be given only steamed or cooked carrots because raw carrots may cause choking. For the older child, however, carrots make a wonderful snack. Supermarkets now sell ready prepared, peeled small carrots in bags. With the exception of beets, carrots contain more sugar than any other vegetable, which explains why children find it to be a satisfying snack eaten raw and a tasty addition to a variety of cooked dishes.

YAMS OR SWEET POTATOES

Yams or sweet potatoes are rich in fiber, complex carbohydrates, calcium, potassium, Vitamin A and C. Despite the name, yams are related to the morning glory family and not the potato (from the Andes). When shopping for yams, choose smooth, hard tubers that are free of many spots, cuts, or bruises. They should seem heavy for their size. Store yams in a cool, dry place, suspended in a wire basket or in an open paper (not plastic) bag. Do not refrigerate, which hardens the yam flesh and degrades its taste. Baked yams are delicious and easy to prepare.

TOMATOES

Tomatoes complement many other foods such as poultry, meats, fish, pasta, pizza, and most other vegetables. Perhaps that is why they are one of the most popular vegetables among Americans. Botanically, the tomato is a fruit, but in 1893, the Supreme Court of the United States, in its wisdom, proclaimed it a vegetable! Whether tomatoes are a fruit or vegetable doesn't really matter; they are a delicious food, especially if grown in your garden.

At one time, fresh ripe tomatoes were my favorite food. They were grown for flavor and I'd enjoy tomato sandwiches, tomato marinated with vinegar and onion, or tomato salad. Anything with tomato made a meal more delicious. Much of this has changed with the selection and cultivation of tomato varieties designed for shelf life, machine harvesting, size and shape for canning, with flavor being last on the scientist's plant design list. The university's plant science department has become an extension of agribusiness. These ubiquitous "cardboard" tomatoes should be avoided, and then industry might get the message that consumers desire flavor along with appearance. Greenhouse tomatoes are distinguished by the part of the stem and leaves still attached when they are sold. These are somewhat more tasty than those artificially ripened with ethylene gas on the way to the market. Try growing your own with your child this spring. The taste of a home grown tomato is a revelation! Next best: organic tomatoes at the Farmers Market. Children love to garden, and those who do are likely to taste and enjoy the fruits of their labor.

Tomatoes that are refrigerated or exposed to temperatures below 55 F lose their ripening potential. If you buy tomatoes slightly under-ripe, place them in a paper bag with an apple or banana and let them ripen at room temperature for a few days. This will enhance their flavor and texture.

When you buy canned tomato products such as tomato sauce, tomato puree, tomato paste, or stewed tomatoes, it is best to choose the "no salt added" brands. The regular cans contain as much as twelve times the sodium of unsalted brands. Avoid tomato juice and V-8 type juices which also contain an enormous amount of salt. Many children develop a rash around the mouth from the peel oils found under the skin of tomatoes. This is due to irritation and is not allergy. To prevent rash, wash your child's face with warm water and a mild soap, such as Dove, to remove peel oil.

Tomatoes are rich in Vitamin C, beta carotene, and potassium. They also contain some zinc, folate, and the phytochemical lycopene. Lycopene, an anti-oxidant carotenoid, and other tomato nutrients may reduce the risk of prostate cancer. Tomatoes may also reduce the risk of stroke in men by as much as 55%. That is because the ingredient, an antioxidant linked to stroke protection, is lycopene. The red color common to tomato, watermelon, grapefruit, and guava signals lycopene (a plant pigment). Lycopene is a potent antioxidant working in the body to counter free radicals that can damage cells and their DNA. This antioxidant may also reduce inflammation and cholesterol, prevent blood clots, and "boost immune function." All studies were done on lycopene rich foods, not as a lycopene pill. To obtain the benefits of lycopene, eat those foods high in lycopene such as tomato puree, marinara sauce, tomato salsa, sun-dried tomato, cooked tomato, tomato paste, raw tomato, cherry tomato, grapefruit, guava, and watermelon.

Vine-ripened tomatoes have a higher lycopene content than tomatoes ripened off the vine. Every vegetable, every fruit, has hundreds of phytochemicals. More reason to increase fruit and vegetable consumption.

The following are of no proven benefit for cardiovascular risk reduction: Vitamin C, Vitamin E, or beta-carotene supplementation, garlic, selenium, and chromium.

GREENS

Green vegetables range in color from light to dark. They can be used raw in salads or cooked into interesting side dishes. They are high in Vitamin A (they contain beta carotene like yellow vegetables), Vitamin C, and folic acid or folate, and they contain significant amounts of calcium and iron. Along with other complex carbohydrates, they are an important component to the healthy diet.

Greens generally used in salads are the crispy iceberg and Romaine lettuces, and softer leaf lettuces, such as butter leaf, red leaf, oak leaf and others. The darker the greens, the more nutrition. Although iceberg lettuce is the number one best seller in the United States, it's the least nutritious variety of lettuce. Romaine and loose-leaf lettuces, for example red leaf, contain more Vitamin A and calcium than iceberg. Butterhead varieties have more iron. Aside from lettuce, other delicious greens to add to a salad are endive, watercress, dandelion, spinach, Swiss chard, and mustard greens.

Greens good for cooking are mustard and beet greens, collard, kale, chard, and spinach. These also add tasty, colorful, textural interest to some casseroles.

Experiment with all these greens. Try the ones you've never tasted. You may discover you've been missing out on some delicious vegetables.

Green vegetables are the most common rejects of young children. If you keep preparing and eating them yourself, your youngsters will gradually accept them as part of the normal fare. Hopefully, the habit will continue into the teenage years, when the independent-minded child excludes anything green and goes on a pizza, soda, potato chip, corn dog, M&Ms, and Top Ramen diet. If your family seldom eats green vegetables, it's never too late to correct poor eating choices and habits.

CRUCIFEROUS VEGETABLES

The name, cruciferous comes from the Latin word meaning "cross," because these vegetables bear cross-shaped flowers. Family members include cabbage, cauliflower, brussels sprouts, watercress, broccoli, horseradish, kale, kohlrabi, mustard, radishes, rutabaga, turnip, Asian and collard greens.

These vegetables contain cancer-fighting compounds called *indoles*. Cruciferous vegetables seem to help protect against cancer of the stomach and large intestine. Studies strongly suggest that these vegetables stimulate the release of anti-cancer enzymes. These enzymes and the antioxidant nutrients, such as carotenoid (beta carotene and Vitamin A) and Vitamin C, help remove free radicals, unstable oxygen molecules that promote cancer. As a bonus, most cruciferous vegetables are good sources of dietary fiber. Kale, collard greens, and turnip greens also supply calcium, while others such as brussels sprouts provide iron. Fortunately most children enjoy broccoli. Experiment with this group of vegetables and introduce them early so your child will develop a taste for these wholesome foods.

ONIONS

Onions rank sixth among the world's leading vegetable crops. They are cousins to garlic, leeks, chives, and shallots. Americans eat 50% more onions today than we did ten years ago. The bulbs now rank just behind potatoes and lettuce as our most popular vegetable. Many onions, like Maui Sweet or red Bermudas, are quite juicy because of their high sugar content. Spanish onions are the largest and range in color from yellow to purple and have a mild flavor. White onions tend to be more pungent than yellows or reds. There are no nutritional differences among these types.

Select onions that feel dry and solid all over, with no soft spots or sprouts. Avoid onions with green areas or a strong odor, which is a sign of decay. Cut raw onions produce volatile compounds that irritate the eyes. To lessen eye irritation, hold onions under cold running water as you peel. Also, if you toss the onions in the freezer for 15 minutes before you cut them, you won't tear up. Cooking onions produces a chemical change that makes them much milder. The heat converts some compounds found in onions into a substance that is 50–70 times sweeter than table sugar! Although onions are not loaded with vitamins, they contain antioxidants called phytochemicals (plant chemicals), that in laboratory tests have blocked the earliest changes in cells that enable tumors to grow. These are mostly sulfur-containing compounds, or organosulfurs, the same ones that irritate your eyes and give onions their sharp taste.

Onions are also reported to lower blood pressure and cholesterol levels and may protect against stomach and esophageal cancers. They are a low-fat food and a great flavor enhancer for potatoes, rice, fish, ground meat, sandwiches, and soup. Virtually every cooking method has been used with onions; however, avoid recipes that call for added fats. Also avoid fried onion rings which are extremely high in both calories and saturated fat. Another favorite to avoid is the high calorie, salty, and fatty onion cheese dips and French onion soup.

GARLIC

Garlic is a close relative of the onion. There is much hype about the medicinal powers of garlic, and health food stores continue to make claims that it protects the heart and is an anti-cancer food. To date, few trustworthy studies substantiate these claims. The National Cancer Institute and other universities are currently studying garlic and onion for such effects. But take heart, garlic still wards off vampires!

Many Latin-American children are introduced to garlic at an early age. It is an excellent taste enhancer and you might want to experiment with it by making salad dressing with garlic vinegar. Place several peeled cloves in a bottle of wine vinegar and let stand for two to three days, covered, and then remove the garlic.

Garlic or onion bread is another favorite. Heat the bread in the oven or microwave and then slice the loaf open. Rub the inside with a halved garlic clove or spread with baked garlic and then toast it under the broiler. If you want to use a mild olive oil or Parmesan cheese on the bread, use sparingly.

FRUIT

The most wonderful thing about fruit is that children adore its sweetness, yet it is extremely healthy. Of course too much of any good thing isn't a good idea, so beware of the fruitaholic, the child who is on a total fruit diet, such as grapes, raisins, and juice! It is not the purpose of this book to review in depth all fruit, but I do want to give you an overview to help you understand why fruit is nutritionally important and should be a part of your child's daily diet.

With a few exceptions, such as avocado, fruit is nearly fat-free. Many fruits, especially apples, are high in cholesterol-lowering and blood-sugar stabilizing fiber and also supply some minerals. Three of the most popular fruits—bananas, pears, and oranges—are loaded with potassium, while berries and dried fruit are rich in iron. Citrus fruits, berries, kiwi, and papaya are rich in Vitamin C. Yellow and orange fruits such as apricots, cantaloupes, peaches, nectarines, and mangoes, are the best sources of beta carotene (Vitamin A) and other carotenoids.

Although grapes are usually not thought of as being especially nutritious, recently a cancer-preventing substance has been found in high concentrations in grapes. This suggests that there may be even more powerful compounds in other natural foods. This finding does not mean that people should eat a lot of grapes to prevent cancer. The overall message is that fruits and vegetables are very useful against disease.

Another health benefit of grapes, *for adults,* comes from drinking wine, which can protect somewhat against heart attacks. In particular, red wine may protect against heart disease by preventing the formation of blood clots that can block arteries.

Don't forget that the whole grape is a common choking food and should not be given to toddlers *under two.*

Prunes are a variety of dried plums. As with other dried fruit, the drying process concentrates the nutrients. First and foremost, prunes are a high-fiber food, containing, ounce for ounce, more fiber than dried beans and most other fruits and vegetables. Over half this fiber is of the soluble blood cholesterol-lowering type. Prunes are also rich in beta carotene and are a good source of B Vitamins, iron, and potassium.

Like other dried fruit, raisins are a concentrated source of sticky-sugar calories, and supply 2 mgs of iron per 2/3 cup. That's 20% of the adult RDA for men and 13% of the adult RDA for women. That's as much iron, by weight, as cooked dried beans or ground beef. For the older child or adolescent raisins is a wholesome snack food. For the younger child, a diet of raisins along with excessive juice and crackers, often causes a skinny child with lots of tooth decay. So save this snack for the older child and don't forget to brush teeth afterwards.

To make a healthy low-fat trail mix, combine raisins with other dried fruit, puffed or shredded wheat cereal, popcorn, and sunflower seeds. Add spiced raisin into low-fat yogurt or add raisins and cinnamon to low fat cottage cheese. Or pack plumped, spicy raisins along with cinnamon into a pita bread pocket for a low-fat "Danish."

Real fruit juice is healthy, especially orange juice, if the very important pulp is not removed. All juices should be consumed in moderate amounts. Juices contain most of the fruit nutrients except for the very important fiber that slows down the absorption of sugar. Beverages labeled "juice" must be 100% juice. *Read the labels carefully!* "Juice blends," lemonade, fruit "punches," "drinks," and "juice cocktails," usually contain little juice, the rest being sugar water. Avoid Hi-C, Tang, Hawaiian Punch, Gatorade, Sunny Delight, V-8 Splash, Tropicana Twisters, fruit soda, and "energy drinks." And don't get your child into the soda habit. Soda is a poor choice because it destroys teeth, and its high phosphate content promotes calcium elimination from your body along with an obesity promoting sugar load. There are 10 teaspoons of sugar in one can of Coke. A growing body needs calcium for strong bone development. Diet sodas are a special hazard and should not be a part of your child's normal diet. Many parents mistakenly choose diet soda over regular soda because they recognize that regular soda is so unhealthy. The important thing to remember is that water is the best alternative. The long term effect of artificial sweeteners has not been adequately studied, in my opinion, and therefore should be avoided by children and teenagers. Let's protect our children from nutritional experimentation!

A juice often overlooked is prune juice. This nutritious juice contains 3 mg of iron or 30% of the RDA for adult men, and 20% for women. A cup of prune juice contains 473 milligrams of potassium, about the same amount as eight pitted prunes. It contains a few more calories than orange juice, 182 calories per cup compared to 110 calories in a cup of orange juice. Don't purchase brands with added sugar. Be careful with any juice because it is a leading contributor to becoming overweight and obese.

When buying fruit, remember that fresh fruit tastes the best. If you are buying fruit to eat today, buy what's ripe. For tomorrow or the next day, look for fruit that needs just a little ripening. To hasten the ripening of pears and peaches, put them in a loosely closed paper bag at room temperature. I usually store them in the trunk of my car for a few days.

Fruit that continues to ripen in addition to peaches and pears: apricots, bananas, cantaloupe, kiwi, nectarines, and plums.

Fruit to buy ripe and ready to eat: apples, cherries, grapefruit, grapes, oranges, pineapple, strawberries, tangerines, and watermelon. Buy Organic when available.

CHAPTER 14

The Older Child's Diet

During elementary school years, children spend far more time away from home. School and outside activities consume a large part of each day. Peers, older children, babysitters, TV, the Internet, and teachers influence your child's development. From these role models children pick up behaviors and habits—eating habits, as well as others. Sometimes parents begin to feel uneasy as they realize they have less control over what their children are doing and eating. With diet, as well as behavior in general, your chances of affecting the outcome will improve if you set a good example at home instead of resorting to criticism and threats.

One area that parents often question me about is school lunches. "What can I prepare for my child to take to school? It must be something convenient, safe, and transportable," they often ask. How can parents also make lunches nutritious and appealing? The latter is essential if you want to make sure your child won't trade the lunch you prepared for a bag of chips and cupcakes!

In my family, we have dealt with the problem of school lunches for years. We have developed some good, nutritious recipes which have passed the test of time as well as the criteria for convenience. "Good food" need not be boring. Children need not feel deprived of life's goodies. Besides fresh fruits and fresh fruit juices, there are lots of nutritious low-salt, low-fat, low-sugar snacks easily prepared and commercially available. I will share them with you in the upcoming pages.

As a parent, you can become an activist whenever you see lots of junk food in a public or private school lunch program or at a PTA and after-school activities. Insisting that fresh fruit be offered alongside the snow cones, candy bars, chips, hot dogs, etc., won't make many inroads without community support. These junk foods are too tempting for most children to resist, and the fruit will be left to rot, especially if it is unripe and tasteless. Your opponents will then remind you that your idealism is "not practical." Don't accept such negativism. Armed with this book, you can explain why wholesome foods are practical, and when properly prepared and presented, are welcomed by children. Most parents realize their obligation to protect their children against the hazards of life. It is time to realize that junk foods are some of these hazards. In order to protect a child from falling into the habit of consuming large quantities of harmful foods, it is best not to have them available except for special occasions.

It is time I told you what I believe junk food is, if you haven't already guessed. To me junk food is that which contains an excess of calories from fat and sugar. In addition, salt is often a major ingredient, and fiber is usually absent or extremely low. It is untrue that "junk foods" are void of nutrients. They often contain many nutrients, including protein, minerals, and vitamins. What makes them undesirable is the imbalance they bring to our diets. Crackers, chips, hot dogs, salami, pepperoni pizza, ice cream, french fries, granola bars, Milky Ways, Lunchables, Hot Pockets and Top Ramen are a few examples of disaster foods, loaded with salt, fats, sugar, and depleted of fiber. If you don't believe that these foods have become the mainstay of our children's diet, look at a typical week's menu from an elementary or high school, public or private, in your community. I'm not suggesting that these foods never be consumed. They can be enjoyed as party or holiday foods. Daily consumption is what makes junk foods dangerous.

When I first began cooking for myself as a graduate student in Philadelphia, the supermarket visit was an adventure in gastrochemistry. What were the food technologists coming out with today? I examined the shelves with the same glee I felt going to attend a yearly new model car show.

Instant rice and instant mashed potatoes. One-minute oatmeal and wheat cereal. Chocolate cake and bake mix in a jiffy. Instant chocolate pudding. All my favorites now at my fingertips! Frozen turkey pot pie, ice cream, and canned peaches for a high living dinner.

Now I'm talking like a traitor about these foods. They did carry me through hard times. The nutritional ravages against my body by my chosen diet were not visible, so who knew? What I didn't realize then is that it isn't significantly more time consuming or difficult to eat healthy foods. It takes only moments to wash a fresh ripe peach or peel an orange.

Like many other physicians of my generation, we smoked cigarettes and overconsumed most of the foods I am now condemning. We were completely ignorant of the connection between diet and what we called degenerative diseases of adulthood, which we believed were inevitable. It wasn't until I completed my formal medical training that I learned about the lipid hypothesis, the Food Industry's corrupting of revered scientists, and how inflammation can be triggered by a sugar and high saturated fat diet.[56] This gradually changed my approach to nutrition from a biochemical concept to actual food choices. It is clear that with all the new nutritional information, our children have an opportunity to enjoy the rewards of improved health and vigor throughout adulthood. As parents, we have the obligation to provide the best we can for our children as well as for ourselves. One does not have to be wealthy to provide the best nutrition. In fact, healthy foods often cost less than many of the expensive processed meals passed off as food.

For those parents who don't want to cook or don't have time to cook there is always "take out," but *avoid fast food take out!* In northern California there are many supermarkets besides Whole Foods that sell wholesome "take out" food choices. They are not inexpensive and unfortunately this eliminates or limits the choices for many low-income families.

BREAKFAST

Many families face a time crunch getting to work or school in the morning. Children often try to capture that last moment of sleep before getting up for school, or teenagers may be more interested in hair or makeup, so there is seldom time for breakfast. It is estimated that 50–70% of students go to school without breakfast and that an adequate breakfast is consumed in no more than 20% of American households. Some youngsters have grown so accustomed to not eating breakfast that they don't feel hungry until midmorning.[57]

So the question comes up—just how important is breakfast? My answer is an unequivocal *very*! Studies on school children show a strong link between a nutritious breakfast and improved school performance. Furthermore, the studies reveal that school performance is adversely affected by omitting breakfast. Children who skip breakfast seem to be more jumpy, have a harder time relating to peers and teachers, and have difficulty concentrating. The physiological reasons for these behavioral changes are poorly understood to date, but repeated observations have made them impossible to dismiss.

It's logical to assume that similar behavior and performance changes occur in adults who do not take the time to eat an adequate breakfast.

For most people the time span between dinner and breakfast is anywhere from eleven to thirteen hours. Omitting breakfast adds another three hours to that fast. Fasting for this length of time puts a stress on the body and causes the formation of fatty acids which are released into the bloodstream. Free fatty acids contribute to the atherosclerotic process that damages and rapidly ages our blood vessels. Fasting also strains the gallbladder, which may lead an adolescent or adult to become more susceptible to a gallbladder attack. It is not my wish to deny the spiritual benefits of fasting to anyone whose religion recommends it for "cleansing the spirit," but there is no scientific evidence to recommend fasting from the nutritional point of view.

Breakfast on the run is one way of dealing with late starters, short of complete behavior modification. By that I mean a glass of 1% fat milk, a banana, and a whole wheat bagel with a wedge of low-fat Laughing Cow Cheese smeared on it! Peel and eat the banana on the way to school. Add a hard boiled egg for more protein. Another alternative is a smoothie—4 oz glass of real orange juice blended with a banana, strawberries, or ripe pears, plus 3 oz of 1% fat milk.

Instant cooked cereal such as oatmeal, cream of rice, quick cream of wheat, Pillsbury Farina, and quinoa may work if one has a little more time. Yes, they are very processed, and because these cereals are so highly processed, the fiber has been milled out, unlike regular oatmeal which contains an appreciable amount of fiber. Replace the fiber by adding fresh fruit, such as blueberries, to the cereal. Remember what we discussed earlier. Until the food industry comes on board, compromise is a must to maintain parental sanity. So add hot water or milk and serve! The protein content of an average serving made with 4 oz of milk is a respectable 8 grams. These cereals are low in fat and high in complex carbohydrates, with no sugar added.

Such cereals as Quaker 100% Natural, Heartland, and some granola are extremely high in fat, sodium and sugar. These cereals boast "naturalness," but oils and sugars have been added—a not so natural occurrence. Since a high fat, high salt, sugary diet is more responsible for malnutrition in America than dietary deficiency, many cereals should be avoided. Read the Nutrition Facts labels on the boxes and select cereals with less added sugar and less sodium and more fiber per serving.

Dry cereals have won a place in the traditional American breakfast. Some observers have stated the nutritional value of dry cereal is proportional to the amount of milk used with each serving. In many instances this is true. However, some of the dry cereals offer better nutrition than others. It is important to read the Nutrition Food label on dry cereals since most overuse simple carbohydrates such as added sucrose, corn syrup, fructose, HFCS, honey, or molasses. Froot Loops, Cocoa Puffs, Sugar Pops, Cap'n Crunch and Honey Combs are but a few of the cereals to avoid. Of the dry cereals, Barbara's Shredded Wheat or high fiber Cranberry, Kashi Go Lean and Heart to Heart are cereals that rate more favorably because most are low sodium, with less simple sugars and have some fiber.

My favorite cereal when I was a kid was Rice Krispies. I loved to read the "comics" on the box: Snap, Pop & Crackle. It is nutritionally one of the worst dry cereals with little to no fiber. The best part of this cereal is when it became a part of one of my favorite chocolate bars: Nestle Crunch Chocolate Bar. One of my many weaknesses. (My wife calls me a hypocrite when she sees me sneak one at the movies!)

Instant breakfast bars are really candy bars masquerading as food. Sports bars contain large amounts of sugar in the form of fructose, honey, molasses, corn syrup, dextrose, maltose, sorbitol, corn solids, and lactose as discussed earlier. Most of these products are 40–70% simple carbohydrate when totaled. Not only do these sticky carbohydrates promote tooth decay, but they provide a high degree of calories without the natural nutrients of real food. Many of these bars are low in fiber, compared with the usual amount of fiber accompanying equivalent calories found in real food. They will push your child closer to an early metabolic syndrome. Their sodium content is often excessive as well. Check nutrition labels for sugars, fat content, and fiber. The Nutrition Facts and ingredients label may be more revealing than the hype on the wrapping. It's true that a child may be eager to eat these breakfast bars, while hot cereal causes a lengthy debate, but the result is an instant poor dietary habit. The next time you're shopping, check the ingredients on the Pop Tart package. The first nine ingredients are sugars and then comes the trace of "dried apples." The low fat variety is an expensive jelly sandwich on toast!

As for pancake mixes, most contain too much salt. It is estimated that three pancakes, about 4 inches in diameter with a patty of melted butter on each, provides 37 grams of fat and well over 1,000 mg of sodium. Pancakes are a favorite for children and adolescents alike. Fortunately it is not hard to prepare a nutritious pancake. Select a low fat, low or reduced salt mix. Many new ones arrive on the shelves monthly. If the recipe calls for milk, use reduced-fat milk. Reduce the suggested oil by a third, and if directions call for an egg to be added, substitute two egg whites and discard one yolk to add extra protein. Use a non-stick un-greased frying pan or griddle.

To make good pancakes, the non-stick pan or grill must be suffi-ciently heated. If it is not hot enough, the pancakes will be tough, since pancakes must be cooked rapidly; however, be careful to avoid making the pan hot enough to burn them. Test the temperature by dropping a few drops of water in the pan—it should sizzle immediately.

A breakfast favorite of mine is *palatschincken*, an Austrian crepe or pancake. It's easy to make. Prepare a low-fat, low-salt pancake mix but add more liquid to thin the mix. Pour about one tablespoon into a hot non-stick pan. Allow it to spread very thinly over an area about five inches in diameter. Turn it over and cook briefly. Remove the thin crepe from the pan and place on a dish. Put a tablespoon of your favorite fresh berries in the middle and roll it up like a blintz or tortilla. Sprinkle with a little pow-dered sugar. Try it on a relaxed Sunday morning. It's especially delicious when it's raining or snowing outside!

CHAPTER 15

More Foods Children and Adults Need

FISH AND SHELLFISH

Tuna, pollack, cod, salmon, and flounder account for at least three-quarters of all the fish Americans eat. Other varieties such as bass, catfish, trout, monkfish, orange roughy, and Mahi-mahi are growing in popularity. Fish provide low cholesterol, low saturated fat, and high protein, and should be consumed more often by children, adolescents, and adults. The greatest downside to fish is that some fish, such as shark and swordfish, may be high in mercury. Another important caveat is that some fish from polluted waters, for example, San Francisco Bay, have stored enough environmental toxins that the San Francisco Public Health has signs at most fishing spots and piers warning against consuming too much of some fish caught in the bay:

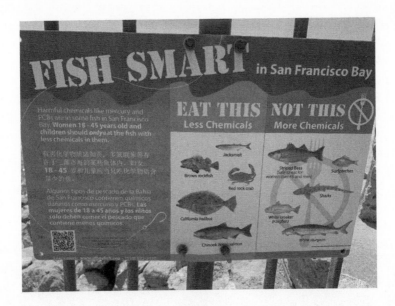

Some children enjoy fish from an early age while others seem to acquire a taste for fish a little later. This may be cultural, since most of my Asian and Hispanic patients seen to enjoy fish and shellfish by one year of age.

Unfortunately, fish sticks, "Fillet O Fish," fish ' n chips, and other types of fried fish appeal to children. Fish sticks are coated with crumbs or batter, fried, and frozen. Because they are easy to reheat in the microwave, they appear to be a simple and nutritious answer to preparing fish. Although fish sticks and these fried fish products are an excellent source of protein, they are made with pollock, an inexpensive fish very low in omega-3 fat. They are often coated with as much as 13 grams of saturated fat or about 45% calories from fat. There's also a lot of added sodium—more than 900 mg per serving in some brands. Add salty ketchup, tartar sauce, or cocktail sauce and you've already exceeded the daily total Nutritional Guidelines recommendation for salt. If you do buy fish sticks, look for brands that say baked low-fat and low-sodium. They should contain four grams of fat per serving or less and half the salt found in regular fish sticks. For example, Mrs. Paul's Low Fat Fish Sticks contain 4 grams of fat and 450 mg of salt per five-stick serving. This is a reasonable compromise if you're looking for something easy to prepare after an exhausting day. *Check the Nutrition Facts label.*

Fish provides more than relatively low-fat protein. It is high in DHA docosahexaenoic acid, which is the fatty acid (a component of fat) that is needed for optimal brain growth and eye development. (Refer to the earlier chapter on nursing and breast milk.). EPA (eicosapentaenoic acid), another fatty acid found in fish, lowers blood cholesterol and protects arterial walls against the harmful effect of LDL cholesterol. These compounds are referred to as omega-3 fatty acids (These "fats" are referred to as "fish oils") and are also found in shellfish.

Another or second variety of omega-3 fatty acid, *alpha-linolenic acid* is found in plant foods and is especially high in oils like canola oil. This essential fatty acid (a fat that the body can't manufacture) is needed for the growth and maintenance of our cells, tissues, and entire body. *Alpha-linolenic acid* is converted to EPA and DHA.

There is another essential fatty acid. It is called *linoleic acid.* Foods high in linoleic acid are vegetable oils such as corn, safflower, soybean, and sunflower seed oils. Most of us eat ten times as much linoleic acid as alpha-linolenic acid. It is believed that the ratio should be closer to 1:1. When linoleic acid dominates too heavily over the omega-3s (alpha-linolenic acid, DHA, and EPA), we may be more prone to illness that causes inflamed muscles and joints, increased menstrual cramps, heart arrhythmias (irregular heartbeats), and even postpartum depression. A 3 ounce serving of baked salmon provides almost 2 grams of EPA plus DHA. That is 10 times the calculated current intake found in the average American diet.

If you don't like fish, substitute your polyunsaturated salad oil (corn, safflower, or soybean oil) with a plant omega-3 oil such as canola oil. Remember, though, it is important to keep total fat low, and if you follow my diet suggestions, you will automatically consume sufficient essential fatty acids or fats.

As much as I believe fish is an important part of the diet, pregnant women should avoid fatty fish such as sablefish, mackerel, bluefish, and stripped bass because they contain pesticides, mercury, and cancer-causing PCB's. Eat salmon instead. A 1994 study of San Francisco Bay waters found unsafe methyl mercury levels in some fish caught there, prompting warning that consumption of these fish be severely restricted. Pregnant women can avoid excess mercury by consuming mercury free canned tuna. Any freshwater fish caught in inland lakes, especially the Great Lakes, are more likely to be contaminated with PCB's and dioxin and should be completely avoided especially during pregnancy. PCB's have been shown to contribute to learning problems in children.

MEATS AND POULTRY

Americans love meat! Meat and poultry are the central focus of most of our meals. Meat is high in saturated fat and cholesterol. In recent years, consumers have been made aware that a diet high in meat is associated with colon and prostate cancer and increases the risk of an early heart attack—the number one cause of death for American men and women. Does that mean you should not eat meat?

Children, adolescents, and adults can nutritionally benefit from a small amount of meat in their daily diet. The emphasis should be on small. For a teenager or adult, no more than a 3.5 oz serving per day. That portion amounts to the size of a deck of cards. Meats and poultry are exceptionally rich in iron, zinc, and Vitamins B-6 and B-12. These nutrients are difficult to obtain in a meatless diet. Choose lean meats.

Pork is not as lean as skinless chicken breast, turkey breast, or fish. However, if you eat small portions and pay attention to trimming away all visible fat, and stay with lean cuts, pork provides many important nutrients. Pork is an excellent source of thiamine, zinc, iron, and high quality protein. Bacon, sausage, spareribs, and hot dogs are extremely high in fat, salt, and nitrites. Ham is also high in salt and nitrites. These nitrites combine with protein during cooking and produce *nitrosamines,* which are linked to stomach cancer. These foods should be reserved for very special occasions and not be daily fare for your children or yourself.

Gourmet sausages are appearing at many markets. Labels that brag "95% fat free" may actually contain many saturated fat grams along with nitrites and a high sodium content. Before buying these tempting delicacies, read the Nutrition Facts label plus the ingredients to get beyond the promotional hype. If you choose to eat them occasionally, be sure to decrease that day's fat allowance in other meals.

3.5 ounces of bacon contains a whopping 1,000mg of sodium! Canned ham, Canadian bacon, and cured ham all contain about 1,000 mg of sodium.

Not all the chicken we eat is low in fat. Eating chicken with the skin will more than double the amount of saturated fat. Chicken skin has 80% of its calories from fat, and over 20% is from saturated fat. Dark meat contains more fat than white meat and is slightly higher in cholesterol as well. Most children love chicken and it is an extremely versatile meat. There are recipe books devoted entirely to chicken. Consult them and don't be afraid to alter the recipes by decreasing or eliminating any added cream, butter, or margarine.

A chicken favorite among children is McDonald's Chicken McNuggets. These nuggets are loaded with 15 grams of mostly saturated fat, with 50% of calories from fat! Conscientious parents who want to give their child "the best of the worst" mistakenly choose McNuggets or the fried fish. A lower fat choice is a hamburger without cheese and a carton of milk instead of the soda. If you must buy the fries, which are loaded with the artery-damaging fats and salt, settle for a small order to share. Of course, fried chicken should be avoided or kept for very special occasions.

Chicken liver is another favorite that should be avoided, even though it is relatively low in fat. The liver is an organ that concentrates all toxins and therefore may contain higher levels of pesticides. Pesticides often contaminate the grains fed to the chickens or seeds eaten by "organic" or free range chickens, since DDT and other pesticides remain in the soil for years.

Turkey breast is the leanest of all meats with 7% of calories from fat. Turkey breast with skin has only 18% of calories from fat. Almost all of the fat in turkey is found in the skin. Dark turkey meat is higher in fat, but is relatively lean if eaten without the skin. Roaster and hen turkeys are good choices for broiling, roasting, or grilling, as they are the most tender. Hens have a larger proportion of white to dark meat. Tom turkeys are larger and older than roasters or hens, and have a reputation for being tastier. Ground turkey is an excellent substitute for ground beef, but it usually needs more seasoning and moisture. Try fresh herbs to add both moisture and flavor. Egg white or tomato juice also enhances flavor and adds moisture to ground turkey. Packaged ground turkey often contains dark meat and may contain more fat. Avoid turkey rolls, and those turkey slices in "convenient" little bags. Instead, choose sliced fresh turkey from your deli. "Lunchables" are to be avoided since they are loaded with salt, and nitrites. There are healthier convenience foods available for your children.

Eating less red meat does not mean your child should eat more chicken or turkey. The most important recommendation for healthy eating is to make vegetables, fruits, and grain products the largest and most appetizing part of your family's diet.

CHAPTER 16

The Adolescent's Diet

The subjects of obesity and eating disorders such as anorexia nervosa and bulimia are extremely important since both often begin before the onset of puberty. However, it is beyond the scope of this book to discuss exhaustively these important problems. I would rather refer you to your physician to direct you to one of the many excellent books available. For older adolescents, a useful formula for calculating ideal body weight based on barefoot height is:

Males: 5 feet = 106 lbs + 6 lbs per additional inch.
Females: 5 feet = 100 lbs + 5 lbs per additional inch.

Adolescence may be defined as the teenage years between 12 and 20, but physical maturation and changes in nutrient requirements actually begin at younger ages and extend into young adulthood. The spurt of growth during adolescence is second only to the rate of growth during infancy, but less predictable. Every parent knows how important good nutrition is for their adolescent son or daughter and naturally turns to authorities such as physicians, dietitians, or "trainers" for guidance. Here is where more confusion begins since nutrient allowances, or Recommended Daily Allowances for adolescents (RDA's) are only estimates or "educated guesses." Nutritionists often take data on young children and adults, and apply it to adolescents without actually measuring their needs. The unusually tall teenager and the early maturer or late maturer will vary considerably in their needs. Their nutritional requirements (RDA's), therefore, should be looked upon more as "guidelines" and not embraced dogmatically. For example, a 14-year-old boy may require 600 to 1200 milligrams of calcium a day, depending on absorption rates of 50% or 25%. The RDA of 1200mg of calcium per day, is thus designed to meet the needs of the adolescent who is growing at the fastest rate. Levels less than that may be quite adequate for many teenagers. This explains the absence of problems in areas of the world where the daily intake is a minimal 200 to 300mg of calcium per day.

Teenagers gain 50% of their bone mass during their pubertal growth spurt, and 90% of total body calcium is found in the skeleton (bones). Because most of a girl's bone mass in the spine and upper femur (thigh bone) is reached at age 16 years, anything that interferes with mineralization of bone during these critical growth years can have long-term consequences. This is the best age to prevent osteoporosis and future broken hips, especially since there are limited treatments for osteoporosis at the present time. It is between ages nine and twenty four that most children store calcium in their bones. These are the years when many adolescent girls favor diet drinks and consume little calcium rich dairy products. Osteoporosis is best prevented by maximizing calcium intake during these years. Encourage your teenager to drink non-fat or 1% milk. Avoid juice unless it is fortified with calcium to get the needed amount of calcium. A Vitamin D fortified calcium supplement may be needed if your child has an aversion to dairy products.

It is sometimes argued that teenage athletes need extra protein, vitamins, or a higher amount of a specific amino acid, like "glutamine." We've all seen the picture of the athlete sitting down to a big steak dinner during training. "Pure muscle building protein" in the form of supplements or meats does not increase strength or help build muscles. Muscle size and strength are developed by muscular work, not by eating meat or magical protein drinks. Extra complex carbohydrates, such as whole grain bread, brown rice, potato, whole grain cereals, pasta, vegetables, and fruit, are desirable to provide the extra energy for the muscular work and growth that go into muscle building. It is also rare for any healthy athlete to need salt tablets as a supplement to compensate for salt lost in perspiration. An exception to this is the teen football player training with the squad after school in 90 degree heat. It's not so much salt as it is water, pure water!

A high protein diet removes calcium from the body. Leading nutritional experts of the World Health Organization recommend progressively decreasing levels of protein to preserve calcium.[58]

Another myth is that beef is the best protein. It certainly is an excellent source of iron, but fish, egg white, breast of chicken, and turkey are equally good sources and considerably lower in fat and cholesterol. Also plant protein from brown rice, quinoa, wheat, beans, and corn are excellent sources of very low fat proteins. Non-fat milk, although often thought of as a "calcium food" is extremely rich in non-fat protein, although low in iron.

Nutritional deficiency of protein, simple carbohydrate, or fat is extremely rare among American teenagers. At highest risk for protein and calcium deficiency are teenagers on extreme weight loss diets, teens from poor families, and those who eat no animal products. The deceptive meat and poultry industry would have you believe otherwise.

Fad diets seem to work—that is, weight is lost. The reason I'm taking time here is because so many teenage athletes are being sold by their coaches many of the bogus concepts detailed in "nutrition" books. Nutritional advice based on the "diet du jour" should be dismissed as yet another untested theory. Most are not sustainable for life, and the fad diet will soon fade into history. Unfortunately, it will probably be replaced by another one filled with exaggerations based on half-truths, pseudo-science, and convincing anecdotes.

Many nutritionists, in their preoccupation with deficiency states, continue to proclaim in the lay and medical literature that fast foods or junk foods allow the vast majority of adolescents to maintain an adequate nutritional status, despite their erratic eating patterns. These nutritionists state that despite the pattern of skipped meals, or choosing pie or fried chicken over lower fat, high complex carbohydrate choices, teenagers will receive the necessary amounts of vitamins and minerals because of the sheer quantity of food they consume. I hope by now the reader will appreciate the absurdity of such notions.

These apologists for the Food Industry claim that the links between salt and hypertension, high fat and cardiovascular disease, gallbladder disease, and some cancers are not conclusive. As an aside, the tobacco industry continues to make similar assertions. There are nutritionists who will tell you to consume all the salt you want, and this advice gets promoted on TV programs such as 20/20. They would have you believe that the major nutritional issues confronting teenagers relate to calcium, iron, and protein or Vitamin A and C deficiency. This is a typical half truth. No wonder parents are totally confused over what constitutes a nutritious diet. Experts, often aligned with the Food Industry, must share the responsibility for this confusion. Because of commercial hype and promotion, many adolescents incorrectly believe that the more protein in their diet the better. But excess protein is not converted to muscle, it's converted into fat! As pointed out earlier, most teenagers need *less* than 60 grams of protein a day (unless pregnant or breastfeeding). While adolescent boys often overdose on protein, I'm concerned about those teenage girls who go in the other direction, under-consuming nutrients, while surviving on no-cal soda, chips, and candy or, "sports" bars.

A 16-year-old who is anxious to "bulk-up" should avoid all those supplements and protein powders, creatine, and taurine, and instead work-out with weights and eat my recommended diet. The slick advertisements found in sports magazines easily seduce teenagers as well as parents into believing the benefits promoted by these multivitamins, minerals, amino acids, protein drinks and powders, etc. Trainers supplement their income by suggesting that these kids need a high protein diet to build muscle because they are growing so rapidly and expending more energy than the average adolescent. The main beneficiaries of supplements sold in health food stores and gyms are the pocket books of the purveyors of these items.[59]

In the United States, fresh fruit is usually available year round, but frozen and canned fruit are also nutritious. Although fruit loses some vitamins during the canning process, the loss is less than found in canned vegetables. This is because fruits are processed at lower temperatures, which destroys fewer nutrients. Try to avoid fruit canned in heavy syrup since it contains fewer vitamins and more sugar calories. Select water-packed canned fruit or canned fruit in unsweetened juice. Frozen strawberries, blueberries, cherries, and peaches are processed without cooking, and therefore there is little nutrient loss.

Dried fruits are an excellent source of vitamins, minerals, and fiber. Dried prunes, raisins, apricots, peaches, and apples are available in most markets. If possible, purchase the no-sulfite-added variety. Mild sulfite sensitivity or allergy may cause a slight tickling of the throat, while severe reactions can result in asthma or breathing difficulty. Check the health food stores for sulfite-free dried fruit. If you're not sulfite sensitive, variety packs that contain sulfites are available in most supermarkets.

Pregnant teenagers have special nutritional needs because there are at least two growing bodies—the adolescent and the fetus. Protein requirements are increased by 10–15 grams per day, bringing the daily recommended protein intake to 60 grams per day. Most women in the United States, including those who might be at risk due to age or socio-economic status, easily meet this level.

"Enzymes," DHEA (sold in many gyms alongside "High Performance" Ultra-whatever bars as a supplement) and "natural" multivitamin mixes promoted by coaches and trainers to the psychologically vulnerable teenagers and their parents, have as much nutritional value as a pla-cebo. "Power bars" are no substitute for real food. The teenager may feel and say, "I took the protein vitamin drink and immediately felt that power surge." But vitamins and minerals do not work that way. What they are reporting is the dramatic placebo effect of suggestion (or perhaps it con-tains lots of sugar and caffeine!).Wishful or magical thinking is powerful and often clouds the intellect. Trainers and gyms often supplement their incomes with the concoctions they sell. Such conflict of interest may get in the way of their usual good judgment. They often give you what I call a "nutrition-biochemistry babble" sales pitch, which sounds very convincing to anyone with a casual understanding of clinical nutrition.

Which brings me to another pseudoscience fad: ginkgo biloba, gin-seng, guarana, chromium picolinate, Vitamin B12, coenzyme Q10, and especially creatine. There is little or no scientific evidence to support the claims made by "health" food sellers for most of these substances. The only pill or drink that will boost your energy is one containing a stimulant, such as caffeine, and the effects of these stimulants wear off within hours.

Ginkgo biloba has been used for centuries in Chinese medicine and its effect on thinking, mood, alertness, and memory have been subject to many studies, but many of these studies have been of poor quality. This is not the way to improve your memory.

Ginseng is a relatively safe herb. It is said to reduce fatigue and en-hance stamina and endurance. Most research concludes it does not im-prove oxygen use or aerobic performance, or influence how quickly you bounce back after exercising. There are many varieties of ginseng. Per-haps the scientists were not using the best or most effective ginseng.

Guarana is an herb that induces a feeling of energy because it is a natural source of caffeine.

Chromium picolinate is a trace mineral widely marketed to build muscle, burn fat, and increase energy and athletic performance. None of these claims are supported by research. Too bad it does not work that way. I sure could use some!

DHEA is marketed as a "fountain of youth," and prevents cancer, heart disease, and infectious disease, among other things. Doesn't it make you want to run out and get some? Unfortunately, the truth is that DHEA has no proven benefits and some potentially serious health risks, such as lowering levels of healthy HDL cholesterol and producing acne, increased body odor, and facial hair in women.[60]

Creatine is another supplement that many of my teenage patients say they take on the advice of their "trainer" to build muscle mass and improve athletic performance. While there are no adverse effects from taking creatine in doses of 2–3 grams per day as recommended on the bottle, there are very few studies of sufficient size and duration to allow confidence about the lack of adverse effects.

It is helpful to inform the athlete that the muscle and strength they are working so hard to gain is being broken down and used as an expendable fuel source. Carbs should be ingested throughout the course of the day, but they are particularly important during the times surrounding athletic activity. Before working out, carbs are important to bolster blood glucose and muscle glycogen stores. Athletes are advised to consume a high carb meal about 3–4 hours before training. That means treating lunch as an important pre-training meal. In addition, a high carb snack should be taken about 2 hours before training (as real food, not a candy "power bar").

If the teenager is a "scholastic athlete," one who trains 1–2 hours a day at least 5 days a week, the post-exercise meal becomes very important in replenishing diminished muscle glycogen. This glycogen is the primary fuel for the next day's workout. This meal is important in keeping muscle from post-exercise breakdown. Maximize the build up of glycogen by providing this high-carb meal with adequate protein from real food as soon as possible following the workout. This increases muscle strength and growth.

Adolescents are quick to accept the disinformation found in some "health" books. Some claim, without any scientific evidence, that eating foods in certain combinations will render them indigestible or non-absorbable, or that "toxins" will form if certain foods are eaten together at different times of the day or night.

Another dietary supplement called L-carnitine that is considered a "body building" compound produces trimethylamine-N-oxide (TMAO) in the gut and may lead to early onset atherosclerosis, heart attack, and stroke.[61]

When megadoses of a vitamin are recommended, beware of side effects. A vitamin given in doses so large that it is unlikely to have been obtained from one's natural diet may act more like a drug. By definition, a megavitamin is a vitamin given in a dose ten times the RDA or more.

If there is a specific defect in a person's body chemistry limiting absorption of a vitamin or preventing normal amounts of vitamins from getting across cell walls into the body tissues, then megadose vitamins may be extremely helpful. Fortunately, most of us do not have these problems.

If you still believe that a high saturated fat/sugar diet and cardiovascular disease is something that only adults should worry about, then read on: In the January 1997 issue of a prominent American Medical Journal, it was shown how a high saturated fat diet is already at work causing artery blockage during early adolescence. Autopsies were performed on 1,079 men and 363 women between the ages of 15 and 34 who died accidentally. The researchers found dramatic differences in the severity of fatty deposits and lesions on the arteries of young people, depending on whether they smoked or ate diets rich in fat and sugar.

What is the typical teenage lunch or snack? A Big Mac, French fries, and a chocolate shake provide 1,000 calories, with 31 grams saturated fat. In addition, the Big Mac has 960mg of sodium, and that doesn't include what is on the French fries. And this doesn't even take into account the high sugar load and negligible fiber. Many school cafeteria lunches are often as bad or worse.

A simple and valid assessment of the nutritional needs of teenagers is that they are similar to those of other ages except for a greater need for calories. Before moving on, a parental alert on caffeine energy drinks spiked with alcohol must be a part of "Nutrition News." These drinks have become extremely popular and are often used at teenage parties to mask effects of the alcohol. Drinkers also drink beer with "energy drinks" and drive under the influence of alcohol because they wrongfully perceive that their judgment and reflexes are normal. The teenager (or adult) who had three alcoholic drinks and an energy drink is at the same level of intoxication as a person who had three drinks, but thinks it's fine to drive.

There are special situations and needs during adolescence. No discussion on teenage nutrition is complete without some relevant information on iron.

Iron deficiency is one of the most widespread nutritional deficiency problems still seen in the United States. Although there is much written about other minerals and vitamins allegedly being in short supply in our diet, iron deficiency remains a real problem in infancy, adolescence, and especially pregnancy. The mineral iron will be discussed in greater depth in the chapter, "Chemicals of Life."

CHAPTER 17

Nutrition 101:
The Chemicals of Life

This primer offers the basics for understanding what infants, children, and adolescents need nutritionally, and what foods will fulfill those needs. Without a basic understanding of the chemicals of nutrition (carbohydrates, protein, fats, fiber, vitamins, and minerals), the important objective of ensuring nutritional well-being could be easily clouded. A knowledge of how dietary chemicals are utilized by the body is important in determining how much of these foods are needed for health and for the restoration of body tissue in stress and disease. For this reason, these chapters on the chemicals of life are included. Readers should keep in mind that research is constantly adding to our knowledge of nutrition and therefore new discoveries may alter some of the information presented in this book. We must always try to keep an open mind and be prepared to change our beliefs when new, scientifically-collected data warrant it.

The much abbreviated information that follows is a crash course in the basics of nutrition. It will help you read food labels and what's between the lines of these labels. It will make you much smarter about food; and if you act on what you learn here, it will help you and your family become healthier.

THE RDA (RECOMMENDED DIETARY ALLOWANCE)

The RDAs are "estimates of amounts of essential nutrients each person in a healthy population must consume in order to provide reasonable assurance that the physiologic needs of all will be met." This is a public health concept, according to Dr. Alfred E. Harper, past chairman of the committee on RDA. "The underlying premise," he states, "is that, since the requirements of individuals are not known, the recommendations must be high enough to meet the needs of those with the highest requirements." For essential nutrients, therefore, the RDA must exceed the requirements of most members of the population.

ENERGY

Our bodies require a certain amount of fuel to operate efficiently and the fuel we run on is energy derived from calories. Many people don't know that the source of energy is nothing more than calories. The amount of calories we need depends primarily upon our height, weight, age, and the type and amount of activity in which we normally engage. If you take in more calories than you can use, your remarkable body converts the excess into body fat and stores it for possible future use. It takes about 3,500–4,000 calories to produce a pound of body fat.

Calories are delivered to the body as sugars derived from carbohydrates, proteins, and fats. Metabolism is the means by which energy is made available to the body. The basal metabolic rate of a person is the amount of calories needed to "run" the body at rest (during sleep). Added to that is the amount of calories to fuel "normal" daily activity and the calories needed to maintain weight and growth. A sedentary person uses fewer calories (energy) than the one in perpetual motion. Infants and adolescents need many extra calories because these ages are times of rapid growth. After age 35 or 40, many adults who do not exercise need fewer calories to maintain weight. In addition, many adults begin to move more slowly and, therefore, find themselves putting on excess weight while consuming the same amount of calories they ate during their more youthful years. If an adult consumes a mere 25 calories a day in excess of need, in 365 days that would add up to about 9000 calories or a two pound weight gain. If this habit continues, in ten years that would translate to a 20 pound weight gain! This is the plight of many once slender young adults, but it also helps to explain why slow-moving children gain weight so easily, compared to the skinny child who is in constant motion and consumes twice the calories.

Too many calories are a major cause of an expanding waistline, especially if those calories are mostly from sugar or high fructose corn syrup (HFCS).

CARBOHYDRATES

The following are extremely important pages on the biochemistry of foods. It is necessary for you to understand these fundamental concepts in order to appreciate how fuzzy nutritional notions can direct you to poor nutritional and dietary choices.

The carbohydrates are called saccharides (compounds made up of sugar). The simplest are the monosaccharides which are also known as simple sugars. Examples of simple sugars are glucose, or blood sugar; fructose, or fruit sugar, the predominant sugar in honey; and galactose, a simple milk sugar. All sugars contain 4 calories per gram.

When two monsaccharides or simple sugars combine chemically, they form a double sugar, called a disaccharide. Sucrose (table sugar), lactose (milk sugar), and maltose (malt sugar) are examples of the most common dietary disaccharides.

The more complex carbohydrates are known as polysaccharides. Their molecules are composed of combinations of monosaccharides or sugar molecules and are very large. Examples are starch, glycogen (animal starch), and cellulose. The complex carbohydrate, starch, is found chiefly in plants like corn, rice, potatoes, yams, and grains. Cellulose forms the cell walls of plants. Cellulose and starch are made up of simple sugars linked together. The linkages are different enough to make starch digestible but cellulose indigestible.

Another class of complex carbohydrates, consisting of "polymers" of monosaccharides, are the oligosaccharides. Oligosaccharides may prove useful as additives to nutritional products such as infant formulas and adult supplements because of their immune properties. Human breast milk, for example, contains 25 different oligosaccharides, which probably function as natural anti-infective agents. There appears to be a correlation between the oligosaccharide content in breast milk and infant immunity at birth. These oligosaccharides may play an important role in protecting the newborn with an as-yet-underdeveloped immune system, and may be the newborns first line of defense against infections.

The simple sugars are absorbed very rapidly from the digestive tract while complex carbohydrates break down slowly during the digestive process, eventually being reduced to the simple sugars. They are then absorbed into the blood stream in their simple form and converted into energy (calories) for the body to "burn" as fuel for activity or to be stored as fat for later use.

From this you can understand the theory of giving juices to provide "instant energy" or the before game carbohydrate-loading meals of athletes as a source of "slow release" energy or fuel during major competitions. Here is some practical information about sugar and carbohydrates. The sugar bowl on your kitchen counter is only the tip of the iceberg.

There are hundreds of forms of sugar hidden in our diet. Punch, apple and orange juice, energy drinks, fresh fruit, ice cream, hot and dry cereals, pies, donuts, cookies, candy, muffins, chili, pizza, Jello, hot dogs, bacon, ham, salami and cold cuts, stuffing, breads, soups, mayonnaise, ketchup, salad dressing, sweetened yogurt, canned vegetables, beans, and virtually all frozen foods contain sugars.

Besides refined cane and beet sugars (common table sugar sucrose), there is refined fructose, which is similar to other table sugars. Fructose, like all carbohydrates, provides 4 calories per gram, but it has special properties that allow it to be metabolized in a different way. We now understand that high fructose corn syrup (HFCS) is harmful. This widely used alternative sugar and corn syrup is used as an inexpensive sweetener in many sodas and baked goods. The average American consumed about 110–130 pounds of sugar per year in 1998. By 2012 that number was 150 pounds of sugar per year! It is estimated that the average American now consumes over 22–28 teaspoons of added sugars a day. This comes mostly from high-fructose corn syrup and sucrose. This represents 18–20% of calories consumed daily in a typical American diet, and that doesn't include the sugar calories from fresh fruit and fruit juices. This high sugar consumption displaces minerals, vitamins, and fiber found in complex carbohydrates. The lost fiber content from these foods promotes constipation and indirectly contributes to other diseases such as diverticulitis and obesity. There is no RDA for sugar. Other sugars used commercially are molasses, maple syrup, honey, dextrose, lactose, levulose, and the "alcoholic sugars" mannitol, and sorbitol.

Nutritious foods such as dried apples, apricots, and prunes, as well as fresh fruit, are all high in sugars. These sugars are also sucrose and fructose, but they are combined with other nutrients such as minerals, vitamins, and fiber. Sucrose and fructose when in refined forms such as juice, or table sugar, whether white or brown, have been stripped of the fiber content and much of their mineral and vitamin content. In addition, these refined, simple carbohydrates don't fill you up like the high-fiber, low-fat complex carbohydrates. Because complex carbohydrates are bulky, you fill up before overeating.

Most of us have experienced the effect from drinking these simple sugars as a "pick-up" when we are tired or hungry. Because they are rapidly absorbed into the bloodstream, the body responds by pouring out insulin to lower the rise in blood sugar. This causes the blood sugar to quickly fall, often at a level below the original amount. Hunger returns along with "the shakes" as body adrenaline is released to counteract the insulin. Besides this rollercoaster effect, there is evidence that the increase in insulin promotes the dietary sugar to be converted into fat. It seems as though it is the fructose sugar that is most harmful to health. Children and adults who consume fructose, the main sugar in sodas, are more likely to have increased belly fat, called visceral fat. Visceral fat is fat that invades the liver, muscles, and the gut area causing the unwanted "pot belly" sometimes referred to as beer belly. There is a relationship between a large belly, insulin resistance, diabetes, and liver and heart disease.

It's important to note that the detrimental effects of fructose as added sugar, including high fructose corn syrup (HFCS), should not be equated with the fructose in fruit. It's difficult to consume excessive amounts of fructose from whole fruits, which are healthy and safe in reasonable amounts.

Sugar promotes tooth decay, especially when consumed between meals as a sticky candy, in raisins, or pastries. Behavior problems such as hyperactivity have been attributed to a high sugar diet, but most studies have not substantiated this association. The contagious enthusiasm of a birthday party or "free time" at school may be the real culprit rather than sugar. It has become much in vogue to blame misbehavior, learning problems, etc., on refined sugar. I suspect in many cases this may be an attractive escape from the responsibility of improving one's home and school structure. Class size and structure may have more to do with "hyperactivity," and "attentiveness" than a sugar diet.

However sugar may be a factor in some children. A parent might swear that when her child was exposed to a particular food, he or she would become hyperactive. A prudent approach would be to avoid the suspected offending food. Skin and blood testing, or sublingual testing has not proved to be of much value.

ADHD is a condition that is increasing. The cause(s) are multifactorial, or caused by multiple factors such as family history (genetics), diet, and many other unknowns. Dr. Benjamin Feingold, a pediatric allergist, suspected that salicylates, a naturally occurring compound present in many fruits, some vegetables, and a number of other foods, plus artificial colors and artificial flavors are causes of hyperactivity. The Feingold Diet was very popular in the 1970s. It eliminates essentially all manufactured baked goods, luncheon meats, ice cream, powdered pudding, candies, soft drinks, and canned fruit drinks. It also eliminates toothpaste, cough drops, and mouthwash. Does this work? It is estimated that about 2–3% of the ADHD population may be helped by this diet.

HFCS, fructose, and simple sugar, also may contribute to sleep apnea, arthritis, high blood pressure, stroke, and increased risk of cancers of the colon, breast, prostate, and uterus.

Sugar has an important place in nutrition when consumed in small amounts. What do I mean by "small?" In 2009, the American Journal of Clinical Nutrition 89:1037 reported on 88,000 nurses who were followed for 24 years. Those nurses who consumed at least two sugar-sweetened drinks a day had a 35% higher risk of heart attack than those who drank less than one a month. Keep that in mind the next time you succumb to your child's pleadings for a Coke.

LIST OF SIMPLE CARBOHYDRATES

Agave	Evaporated cane juice
Sucrose	Corn syrup
High Fructose Corn Syrup (HFCS)	Maple syrup
Glucose	Molasses
Fructose	Honey
Dextrose	Syrup
Invert sugar	Corn sweetener
Brown sugar	Orange juice concentrate
Grape juice concentrate	Apple juice concentrate
Table sugar	Raw sugar

EXAMPLES OF FOODS HIGH IN SIMPLE CARBOHYDRATES

Berries	Bananas
Oranges	Grapefruit
Apricots	Apples
Melons	Orange juice
Grapefruit juice	Apple juice
Apricot nectar	Peach nectar
Kool Aid	Lemonade
Energy drinks	Hi-C
Tang	Hard candy
Coca-Cola	Soda
Sports drinks	Energy drinks

The foods containing complex carbohydrates have a small percentage of fat and protein in addition to starch and cellulose, the indigestible cell walls of plants. Remember that when you eat rice, corn, potato, or pasta, you are not eating pure starch. For example, buckwheat is fiber rich and high in copper and magnesium while wild rice has more zinc than any other grain. Barley is a good source of fiber and iron, while brown rice is the only rice that contains Vitamin E. These foods contain significant protein with minimal fat, as long as you don't douse them with butter, margarine, oil, or cream. If you must use a "flavor enhancer," use an herbal low-fat sour cream or something similar to "I Can't Believe It's Not Butter." Fresh salsa is another delicious and nutritious topping.

PROTEINS

Proteins differ from carbohydrates and fats chemically in that they contain nitrogen. The proteins of our bodies are composed of twenty-two amino acids, in varying combinations. Of these, eight can't be made by our bodies and are therefore called essential amino acids. These amino acids must be obtained in adequate amounts from the food we eat. They are tryptophan, leucine, isoleucine, lysine, valine, threonine, phenylalanine, and methionine. All eight amino acids must be present in order for a protein to be nutritionally complete. Proteins that contain the essential amino acids in adequate quantities are called complete proteins. Examples are egg white, fish, meat, poultry, and certain vegetables such as soybean and peanut.

Our bodies digest protein to form amino acids. Amino acids are necessary for growth, repair, and maintenance of our body tissues. We need a basic minimum of protein to remain in "positive nitrogen balance." That is, we need to have enough protein intake to balance what our body wears out or excretes. If you are in "negative nitrogen balance," it means that you are excreting more nitrogen (protein) than you are consuming. Your body must then obtain nitrogen by breaking down your muscles and the cells. This is extremely unhealthy and is called starvation!

How digestible a protein is, especially a plant protein, determines how much of its amino acids are actually available to our bodies. Whole proteins must be digested to amino acids before being absorbed into the bloodstream from the intestines. The term "biological value" is used to describe proteins as complete or incomplete. Complete proteins of high biological value are found in meats, egg white, fish, poultry, edamame (fresh soybeans), and nuts. The proteins that do not supply the essential amino acids, or else supply inadequate amounts, are known as incomplete or inadequate. They are usually of vegetable origin and that is why vegetarians should eat a greater quantity or variety of plant proteins. Having said this, I will reiterate that protein deficiency is not a nutritional problem in America. Nutritionists point out the need for increased protein intake during periods of the life cycle when rapid growth takes place. These are infancy, teenage years, and pregnancy. However, protein from meat intake in America is in such excess that we see more of the toxic effects of too much animal protein than protein deficiency.

For example, infants are occasionally fed cow milk which has 20% protein, far in excess of the more nutritional 7% protein of human breast milk. Adolescents often take protein drinks believing that this will increase their muscle bulk and strength. This poor nutrition is not only unnecessary, but potentially dangerous. Too much protein also results in increased loss of minerals, such as calcium.

The RDA for protein for a growing male adolescent who is tall and well developed is 56 grams a day. For those nutritionists who refer to the RDA as a guide, use caution. The National Research Council suggests that a diet should not be considered inadequate if it does not meet the recommended levels.

For those individuals not in a rapid growth phase or not pregnant, 10% of calories is sufficient protein. Pregnant and nursing mothers need extra protein but not nearly as much as some nutritionists recommend. The RDA suggests 74 grams of protein for a pregnant woman and 64 grams for a nursing mother. Remember, this is a very high value and may be extremely inappropriate and excessive for a 5-foot-tall 108-pound woman. For this reason it is more accurate to calculate protein needs using height and body build plus percent of total calories needed, as well as state of health. Few parents will tax their math skill to determine protein needs, and indeed, they shouldn't. In the real world, nobody does this. I do not want to stress numbers, since they will soon be forgotten and are irrelevant to the shopper, who shops for food, and should rely on principles, such as buying fresh produce, whole grains, avoiding high fructose corn syrup, sugar (HFCS) cakes, cookies, and sugary drinks along with high saturated fat protein foods. The at-risk population for protein deficiency is the teenage girl on a diet soda and candy bar diet or the pregnant teenager. These children need special attention and nutritional counseling.

Since 1983, I have worked as a pediatrician in many Central and South American countries as well as in Asia and Africa with a medical organization. My responsibility was to examine each child selected to have cleft lip or palate surgery, and be certain that the child is healthy enough to undergo this surgical procedure and to care for them post-operatively in the recovery room immediately and to be certain that each child receives proper care during their convalescence.

I will never forget the first time I witnessed the devastating effects of protein deficiency. We just completed reconstructing this beautiful six-month-old infant's cleft lip. She was slightly anemic. What I didn't realize was that the infant's poor and uneducated parents were feeding their daughter an infant formula they made with a little milk formula, and extended with mostly cooked corn meal. This is a common practice, since commercial baby formula is expensive, and mothers are not encouraged to breastfeed. Corn is an incomplete protein because it does not contain the essential amino acid tryptophan. As a result, the child was protein deficient, and because I was unaware of her diet, I permitted the surgery to take place. When the baby's sutures were removed at the usual time, healing had not occurred and the beautiful repair fell apart. That moment was the beginning of my interest in earnest with nutrition.

Inadequate intake of essential amino acids over an extended period of time causes "protein starvation" and the protein deficiency disease- kwashiorkor results. Kwashiorkor is an African name that describes affected children with characteristic red hair, swollen bodies, and potbellies. I've seen kwashiorkor many times since that episode in Honduras and other developing countries where poor mothers feed their children formula made from corn instead of breastfeeding. This is a third-world disease and is extremely rare in the United States where over-consumption of protein is the rule.

If one is a vegetarian, or especially vegan, who does not eat any egg white, dairy, or fish, the selection of foods is much more crucial.

True malnutrition rarely occurs in the United States but, if it does, it is usually because of ignorance, or due to a psychotic parent or caretaker. In Marin County, California, there was such a family who provided a low-fat, low-carbohydrate, low-protein vegan diet to their five children. When one died, an autopsy revealed the baby to have severe rickets.

The other children were inspected by CPS (Child Protective Services). The children were found to be emaciated and developmentally delayed, with bony malformations. They were immediately transferred to UCSF Medical Center and were found to have advanced severe rickets due to extremely poor nutrition, lack of Vitamin D in the diet, plus little sun exposure. I saw them 18 years later while working for the California

Children's Services (CCS) as a medical consultant. Remarkably they were completely rehabilitated!

FATS (LIPIDS)

The broad category of chemicals with greasy properties, such as fat (triglycerides), fatty acids, and cholesterol are classified as lipids. The chemical composition of fats is similar to carbohydrates, but one gram of fat produces a hefty 9 calories, over twice the calories obtained from one gram of protein or sugar. The fats in fatty tissue (adipose tissue) are called triglycerides. Triglycerides are one of the three parts of cholesterol in the body: low-density lipoproteins (LDL), high-density lipoproteins (HDL), and triglycerides. When we eat calories in excess, particularly carbohydrate, the body transforms these carbohydrates into glucose. Glucose is then used by the body for energy. However, not all glucose is used. Some forms are transferred to the liver where glucose is converted into glycogen ("animal glucose"), which is then stored in the muscles. Excess glycogen is moved back from the muscles to the liver and the glycogen becomes triglycerides, which are stored in the blood stream. The triglycerides in the bloodstream are milky and fatty in nature. The blood can more easily clot and cause a blockage in your bloodstream. This can lead to dangerous side effects, such as inflammation, heart attack, or stroke. As you can see, it is important for good health to keep your triglyceride levels low. A diet high in refined sugar, especially fructose, raises triglycerides.

This body fat (triglycerides) breaks down into glycerol and three fatty acids. Glycerol can then be converted into sugar and used as body fuel. The fatty acids come in many different lengths and levels of saturation. Saturated fatty acids are opaque at room temperature and are mainly derived from animal sources. Examples of foods which contain predominantly saturated fatty acids are whole and 2% milk, cream, ice cream, cheese, butter, beef, lamb, pork, coconut, coconut oil, and palm oil. Fatty acids (fats) that are liquid at room temperature are usually more "unsaturated." Monounsaturated fats (olive oil, canola oil, avocado), seem to be healthier than saturated fat. When monounsaturated fat replaces saturated fat in the diet, it has a blood cholesterol lowering effect (lowers LDL cholesterol levels).

But can olive oil be used in baking? Some olive oils, such as regular, highly processed olive oil, have a very mild flavor in contrast to extra-virgin and virgin varieties. Olive oil may be used in place of butter or other solid fats in the baking of cakes, cookies, muffins, and quick breads. It doesn't work well for pastries or crusts, because olive or any other oil saturates the flour and makes the finished product dense instead of light and flaky.

Polyunsaturated fats (soybean oil, corn oil, safflower oil) appear to cause less damage to arterial walls than saturated fats, unless they are hydrogenated to make them a solid fat such as stick margarine or Crisco. Hydrogenated polyunsaturated fats contain what is called "trans" fat and are more damaging to your arteries than saturated animal fat such as bacon grease, butter, or cream. Trans fats are found in foods such as French fries, Oreo cookies, pie crusts, chicken pot pie crust (one of the worst foods!), potato chips, and many other foods that may be labeled, "cholesterol-free." Fish fried in melted Crisco or stick margarine along with tater-tots and chicken nuggets may be loaded with artery clogging trans fat. Look at the Nutrition Facts label. Trans fats are now required to be listed on the Nutrition Facts label. Many fast food restaurants have recently removed trans fats from their cooking oil. Foods can call themselves "trans fats free" even if they contain up to a gram of trans fats per serving. If a food contains partially hydrogenated oils, it contains trans fats.

The best way to reduce your triglycerides is to lower simple carbohydrates in the diet. Another way to reduce triglyceride levels is to consume more fatty fish, such as salmon or trout. Taking a daily supplement of fish oil may also reduce triglyceride levels.

In addition, oils are available in two forms: combined oil is in the seed or fruit (avocado) as grown. Free oil can be expressed, bottled, and sold. Corn oil, safflower, and sunflower seed oils are all free oils. Combined oil has the vitamins, minerals, fiber, and other nutrients. To obtain free oil from corn, many kernels must be pressed to get one ounce.

Cholesterol is a lipid or fat-like substance which is found in all animal meat, whole and low fat milk, cheese, butter, liver, sweetbreads, eggs, shrimp, crab, and shell fish. Cholesterol is not found in any vegetables. All those "cholesterol free" advertisements stamped on vegetable oils and margarine are deceptive in that they suggest "healthy," or that somehow the cholesterol was removed. As you will learn, trans fat and saturated fats are far more artery clogging (atherogenic) than cholesterol. Fats in combination with cholesterol are especially atherogenic (bacon and eggs; lobster dipped in butter or melted stick margarine). Boiled shrimp dipped in a non-fat cocktail sauce is a delicious low fat dish and as long as the shrimp is not sautéed or fried, its small amount of cholesterol is of little nutritional consequence.

We have learned in recent years that there are various types of cholesterol, defined in terms of the types of protein they are associated with in the body. Since cholesterol, in pure form, is insoluble in water and blood, it tends to hook up with proteins forming what is called lipoprotein. This is the form in which cholesterol travels in the blood stream.

The body is able to make cholesterol, mainly in the liver, intestinal mucosa (lining), and various body tissues. Some ends up as low density lipoprotein (LDL) and some as high density lipoprotein (HDL). It is primarily the LDL of cholesterol that is most artery clogging (atherogenic) and lead to atherosclerotic vascular disease (heart attacks, strokes, blocked arteries) and that is why LDL is often referred to as the "bad cholesterol." High density lipoproteins (HDL) actually appear to protect against the build up of artery clogging "plaques." HDL (high density lipoproteins) provides a mechanism for removal of excess cholesterol from the bloodstream. HDL cholesterol is often referred to as the "good cholesterol." Aerobic exercise, and substitution of monounsaturated fats for saturated fats raises the good HDLs. (Use olive oil or canola oil instead of butter, margarine, shortening, lard, coconut oils, or hydrogenated polyunsaturated fats).

Small amounts of fats in our diet are important because they contribute a necessary source of flavor. Dietary fat has an essential physiologic role. It delays emptying time of the stomach, thereby delaying the onset of hunger, stores energy, and is part of every cell membrane. In the gut, certain vitamins are absorbed from fats. Cholesterol is important in bile formation (needed for digestion), adrenal, and sex hormones, and has many other important functions such as brain growth. The body can manufacture cholesterol and most fatty acids. Fatty acids not synthesized by our body must be obtained from our food. These are called essential fatty acids. The three fatty acids known to be essential for complete nutrition of infants, children, and adults are linoleic acid (also referred to as omega-6 fatty acids), linolenic acid (referred to as omega-3 fatty acids), and arachiodonic acid (another omega-6 fatty acid). The reason essential fatty acid deficiency is extremely rare is that diets as low as eight percent fat carry no risk of fat deficiency disease!

There are some fatty acids found in fish, such as salmon, called DHA (decosahexaenoic acid) and EPA (eicosapentaenoic acid) which are anti-inflammatory and which may provide a protective effect against the formation of artery blocking cholesterol plaques. They seem to be especially important for brain development during infancy. DHA is found in breast milk and it has recently been added to commercial baby formula because of its reported IQ-enhancing effect. My mother was correct when she referred to fish as "brain food."

It is common to hear supposedly well-informed individuals announce their "low cholesterol levels" as a badge of honor. (Normal healthy total cholesterol ranges between 125mg to 165mg).[62] How naive it is for adults or children to assume that they can consume all the fried eggs, ice cream, tater tots, sausage or hot dogs, potato chips, and French fries they desire because they are "thin" or their cholesterol level is low. A diet high in saturated fats, salt, and highly refined carbohydrate (sugars), regardless of one's blood cholesterol level, will make one more likely to develop bowel cancer,[63] hypertension, gallbladder disease, chronic constipation, and adult onset diabetes (type II).

Adult onset diabetes is often referred to as Non-Insulin-Dependent Diabetes Mellitus or Type-2. People with diabetes have difficulty removing the sugar or glucose from their blood. After we digest a meal, glucose (blood sugar) is produced. In response, the pancreas then secretes insulin, a hormone that enables glucose to pass into the cells, where it is stored as fat or burned as body fuel. In adult onset diabetes, insulin is produced, but it loses its effectiveness and is unable to adequately remove enough glucose from the bloodstream. Overweight and under active people who have a familial history of diabetes seem to more readily develop this insulin resistance or Type-2 diabetes. Exercise and weight loss help prevent the onset of this type of diabetes.

Type I Diabetes is often referred to as Juvenile Diabetes. In Type I Diabetes there is little or no insulin because most of the insulin producing pancreatic cells have been destroyed by something, perhaps a virus. It is unclear what this or these agents are, but the illness is different than the more prevalent Type-2.

In insulin resistant Type-2 diabetes, a diet high in saturated fat and refined sugar is especially dangerous because these diabetics are at great risk for developing atherosclerosis and a heart attack. In an effort to keep the body's blood sugar normal, lots of insulin is secreted. As a side effect, the body's triglycerides rise (blood fat), LDLs ("bad cholesterol") rise and the HDLs ("good cholesterol") fall. Heart disease begins along with stroke, kidney failure, and blindness . . . all part of the disease. Most adults can prevent or delay the onset of these complications by following the dietary advice given in this book. By getting more exercise, eating less saturated fat and protein, increasing complex carbohydrates and fiber, avoiding sugary foods and drinks, you will not only extend your life, you will improve life's quality and better enjoy your children and grandchildren.

Higher consumption of sugar-sweetened beverages by children 12–18 years old is associated with the consumption of foods that are a top source of saturated fat, such as pizza, cakes/cookies/pies, fried potatoes, and sweets! This is the diet that leads to the onset of type 2 diabetes mellitus.

FIBER

What grandmother referred to as "roughage" is now called fiber. Until recently it was believed that fiber had no nutritional value. In fact, food processors removed the fiber from grains such as wheat and rice to "improve" textures and color. They called this refining, which gave flour the smooth white color and texture for our cakes, breads, and cereals.

Bran is often used synonymously, but incorrectly, with the term dietary fiber. Dietary fiber is that part of cereal grains and those vegetables not digested or absorbed by the intestines. Fiber can be divided into two broad categories, soluble (as found in oat bran, barley, beans, carrots, peas, sweet potatoes, yams, and fruit pectin from apples and grapefruit) and insoluble. The insoluble coarse fiber (as found in wheat bran, Kellogg's All-Bran, corn, black-eyed peas, figs, and berries) helps move food through the digestive tract by stimulating the lining of the gut to secrete water and mucus, which softens the stool, making it easier to pass. Soluble fiber can boost stool bulk by absorbing water. Not all soluble fiber gets the job done. Psyllium, the key ingredient in Metamucil holds water the entire way through the intestines and is safe and effective.

Most plants contain both types in varying amounts, but certain foods are particularly rich in one or the other. Whole grains are quite complex and contain substances we know little about nutritionally. Besides minerals such as selenium, copper, magnesium, Vitamin E, phytic and phenolic acids, there are lignins, phytoestrogens (plant estrogens) antioxidants, and other unknown factors. The best way to get fiber plus these other nutrients is to eat a diet rich in complex carbohydrates. Seeds and nuts are also excellent sources.

Now we know that in addition to preventing constipation, insoluble fiber may inhibit the development of colon and rectal cancer, reduce the likelihood of gallstones and decrease the risk of diverticulosis.

Diverticulosis is a condition in which tiny pouches, called diverticula, form within the wall of the colon. When the pouches trap food, they may become painfully inflamed (diverticulitis), causing pain, bleeding, flatulence, diarrhea, or constipation. Experts estimate that, in North America, a third of people over 45 and two-thirds of those over 85 have it. By reducing constipation, the insoluble dietary fiber may help to prevent the development of diverticula and relieve the inflammation once it occurs. Soluble fiber improves blood sugar in adult-onset diabetes and type I diabetes by slowing the absorption of sugar in the intestines, thus reducing the need for more insulin. Soluble fiber also reduces blood cholesterol by lowering LDL ("bad cholesterol").

What isn't clear is whether it's the fiber alone that causes the benefits attributed to fiber. Those adults who consume 25–30 grams of fiber a day, in study after study, have reduced the risk of cancer, heart attacks, diabetes, and the symptoms of diverticulosis. It is assumed that this is because of the fiber in the diet, but it may be the fiber plus the ingredients found in high fiber foods (grains, vegetables, and fruit). Isolating a single ingredient, like fiber or beta carotene, and giving it as a supplement, in the form of a capsule, has yielded disappointing results. There is something about eating whole foods in the form of whole grains, fruits, and vegetables that scientists have not unraveled. That is one reason why I do not encourage the fad of sprinkling bran over your food. In fact, one of the more common causes of recurrent belly pain in childhood is caused by bran (bran-bellyache).[64]

Look for cereals that are whole grain and high in fiber. Avoid the sugar-added cereals. This was difficult to tell until we got the new Nutrition Facts label that now lists *added* sugar in addition to Total Sugar. (See page 166 for a generic example of the new Nutrition Facts label.)

Although there is no RDA for fiber, the recommended intake is 0.2 grams of dietary fiber per pound to a maximum of 35 grams daily. To calculate the recommended dietary fiber for a 25 pound child: 25 X 0.2 = 5 grams of dietary fiber. For a 50 pound child, it would be: 50 X 0.2 = 10 grams of dietary fiber. Or, for a more rapid calculation: for every 25 pounds of body weight, 5 grams of fiber is recommended. Thus a 75 pound child's recommended dietary fiber intake is 15 grams.

EXAMPLES OF CEREALS HIGH IN FIBER

One easy way to select a dry cereal for your children is to have them choose a cereal they like as long as it has at least 3 grams of fiber. Most cereals that have 3 grams of fiber are nutritious.

EXAMPLES OF HIGH FIBER LOW CALORIE FOODS

FOOD	SERVING SIZE	FIBER (GRAMS)	CALORIES
Figs	3.6		190
Dried Figs	3.0	3.6	190
Apple	1.0	3.5	81
Pear	1/2 (large)	3.1	61
Carrots	2/3 cup	3.0	32
Strawberries	1 cup	3.0	45
Broccoli	2/3 cup	2.9	26
Spinach	2/3 cup	2.8	28
Orange	1.0	2.6	62
Zucchini	2/3 cup	2.4	15
Prunes	2.0	2.0	40
Blueberries	1/2 cup	2.0	39
Peach	1.0	1.9	37

If the label says whole grain or whole wheat, it is a whole grain.

If the label says cracked wheat, "made with whole grain," multi-grain, oat bran, oatmeal, pumpernickel, seven-grain, seven-bran, nine-grain, etc., stoned wheat, wheat, wheat-berry, whole bran, it's mostly refined grain.

VITAMINS

Vitamins are organic compounds that cannot by synthesized by our bodies and are necessary in minute quantities in our diet to keep the body in good condition.

If our bodies were maintained by a diet containing only purified proteins, carbohydrates, fats, and the necessary minerals, it would not be possible to sustain life. Vitamins are necessary as an accessory food factor. They act as biocatalysts within the body. That is, they promote necessary chemical reactions in the body, without being consumed in the reactions. They function as co-enzymes or parts of co-enzymes. For the vitamin to work, it must first enter a cell in the body and combine with a particular kind of protein called an apoenzyme. When a co-enzyme attaches to an apoenzyme, a complete or holoenzyme is formed. Extremely small amounts of vitamins are needed. Once all the apoenzymes in the body are saturated to form complete enzymes, more vitamins will collect in the body fluids and be stored, or the excess will be excreted. The vitamins are generally divided into two major groups: fat-soluble and water-soluble. Fat-soluble vitamins are usually found associated with the lipids (fats) of natural foods. These include Vitamins A, D, E, and K. The water-soluble group includes Vitamin C, folate, and the vitamins of the B complex.

The RDA for a vitamin is enough to saturate our entire body with that vitamin. Unlike water-soluble vitamins, the fat-soluble vitamins are stored in our body fat and can be toxic if large amounts build up. So again, we are reminded that too much of a good thing can be harmful. Or, if not harmful, then wasteful since in a normal person most of the water soluble vitamin supplements wind up in the toilet.

Many diseases of mankind, including beriberi, scurvy, night blindness, and pellagra, are known to be caused by lack of these essential food factors. These vitamins were originally assigned letters of the alphabet. Now that we have been able to identify the chemical structures of vitamins, nutritionists prefer to use their chemical names rather than the letters. In some cases, the letters formerly assigned to the vitamins have been dropped entirely. Biotin has been substituted for Vitamin H. Folic acid has been substituted for Vitamin M.

WATER SOLUBLE

Vitamin levels for the water-soluble vitamins are measured in either milligrams (mg, thousandths of a gram) or micrograms (mcg, thousandths of a milligram).

The vitamins of the B complex[65] and their synonyms are listed with the accepted current name first and the historical names in parentheses.

1. Thiamin (Vitamin B-1, antiberiberi substance, antineuritic vitamin, aneurine)
2. Riboflavin (Vitamin B-2, lactoflavin)
3. Niacin (Vitamin B-3, P-P factor of Goldberger, nicotinic acid)
4. Pyridoxine (Vitamin B-6, rat antidermatitis factor)
5. Pantothenic acid (Vitamin B-5, filtrate factor, chick antidermatitis factor)
6. Lipoic acid (thioctic acid, acetate replacement factor)[66]
7. Biotin (Vitamin H, anti-egg white injury factor)

8. Folate (liver lactobacillus casei factor, Vitamin M, fermentation residue factor, pteroylglutamic acid, folic acid group)
9. Inositol (mouse anti-alopecia factor)
10. Para-aminobenzoic acid; PABA
11. Vitamin B-12 (cyanocobalamin, cobalmin, antipernicious anemia factor, extrinsic factor of Castle)
12. Ascorbic Acid (Vitamin C)
13. B Complex group

FAT SOLUBLE

Vitamin levels for the fat-soluble nutrients A, D, E, and K are measured in international units (IUs).

Vitamin A (retinol)

Vitamin D (calciferol)

Vitamin E (tocopherol)

Vitamin K

Vitamins act both independently and often together. Most vitamin deficiency disease is seen predominantly in areas of the world where war and famine exist, and the cases usually show mixed deficiency. It is more common for isolated deficiency to occur in specific circumstances. For example: Vitamin K deficiency as an isolated event occurs in early infancy. The infant most vulnerable is the breastfed newborn. Normal adults rarely lack Vitamin K. In the newborn, however, the quantity of the vitamin derived from the mother is small. At birth the intestines do not contain the bacteria necessary to manufacture Vitamin K and the breast milk does not supply it. Mild Vitamin K deficiency in the newborn is common. Very low levels, as a result of the deficiency, may cause hemorrhages in the newborn. This disaster can easily be prevented by giving the infant oral or intramuscular Vitamin K once soon after birth.

Another situation is found with Vitamin D, the "sunshine vitamin" deficiency. There is a saying in the Alps of Austria, "Fall baby—spring rickets!" Austrian winters are long and cold. Infants are wrapped and away from sunlight from October until late March. The result is that eight months after birth, the infant has soft bones and the extreme irritability which mark rickets. Most of the infants who become deficient are fed cow milk which has no Vitamin D. Human breast milk is also deficient in Vitamin D, but the illness is rarer in breastfed infants. Ironically, the deficiency is also seen in the Caribbean where it is common practice in some cultures to wrap infants completely to keep them protected from the sun.

Vitamin deficiency is very rare in the United States because fresh vegetables are readily available year round. In addition, bread, flour, cornmeal, corn grits, macaroni, and spaghetti products as well as infant cereals and dry cereals are vitamin enriched. In spite of this, there remains a vulnerable group that still exists in this country.

At risk is the person on a high-level macrobiotic diet whose diet is not varied but consists mostly of rice. Beware of bizarre fad diets, regardless of how eloquently they are presented.

Another at-risk group, is the elderly bachelor or widower who may prepare his own foods. Both are particularly prone to the development of Vitamin C deficiency, a syndrome termed "bachelor scurvy." They're not eating enough fruit. Food faddists who avoid raw foods, particularly fruits and vegetables, are at risk to develop Vitamin C deficiencies. Deficiency malnutrition is common among alcoholics, the poor, the elderly, and the chronically ill. In contrast, vitamin excess is a disorder of the well-to-do.

A megavitamin is a vitamin given in a dose ten times the RDA or more. If there is a specific defect in a person's body chemistry limiting absorption of a vitamin or preventing normal amounts of vitamins from getting across cell walls into the body tissues, then megadose vitamins may be extremely helpful. There are, for example, infants born with defective apoenzymes or inborn errors of metabolism. By giving such a patient megadoses of a vitamin you can force the co-enzyme (vitamin) reaction by mass action. Vitamin D resistant rickets is one example where megavitamins can be used to good advantage. Folate or folic acid as a 1mg to 10mg (1,000 micrograms to 10,000 micrograms) daily megadose supplementation before pregnancy may prevent certain types of cleft lips and palates and is currently under investigation.

Claims that niacin regulates blood sugar and is useful in the "megavitamin treatment" of schizophrenia or that it is of value in the prevention of heart problems have not been substantiated by adequate controlled studies. Instead, what we have mostly are testimonials by people, including physicians, that they "felt better" after taking megadoses of these vitamins. It is important to keep in mind that these feelings are based far more on faith and wishful thinking than on scientific fact. The same is true for megadose therapy of vitamins and minerals to correct mental retardation or autism. When faced with a situation believed to be "hopeless," most of us are tempted to try anything as long as it is not harmful.

The usual feeling is, "What do I have to lose, anyway?" In such a case, the decision must remain a personal one. But, be careful. Some of these concoctions are not without danger. Hope should never be taken away from anyone in a desperate situation, but false hope can only lead to disillusionment. When someone realizes he has been "used" or "taken" by a professional opportunist during a vulnerable moment in his or her life, it magnifies the feelings of sorrow and loss.

Consumers are receiving an unprecedented flood of information, some of which is properly analyzed while some is widely publicized without proper scrutiny. This often misguided nutritional information is actively promoted especially by "health food stores" and by doctors who practice unconventional or "fringe" medicine. The Internet is loaded with these "nutritional" promotions. *Caveat emptor*—buyer beware!

The idea that "natural" vitamins provide special benefits for our bodies has been promoted by manufacturers and retailers of these vitamins. vitamins have the same properties whether natural or synthetic. Many vitamins labeled natural or organic are not what you might imagine those terms to mean. Rose hips Vitamin C tablets are made from natural rose hips, which have natural Vitamin C combined with chemical ascorbic acid, the same Vitamin C used in standard tablets. If no Vitamin C were added to the tablet "it would have to be as big as a golf ball." Makers of "natural" Vitamin C often suggest that synthetic vitamins do not contain the hidden or not well-known micronutrients that are included in the natural forms. They point to the "associated factors," flavonoids, proto-pectins, and minerals of the whole fruit, including the so-called "P" factors. Although the rational conclusion is to eat the entire fruit or vegetable to obtain all the nutritional value, consumers are told their diet needs a promoted supplement. Natural B complex vitamins are mostly synthetic chemicals added to yeast and other bases. Vitamin E products are derived from vegetable oils, but in order to concentrate the vitamin in a capsule, various chemical solvents must be used. The vegetable material may be grown with the usual pesticides and chemical fertilizers. Finally, the gelatin capsule must contain a preservative so that it won't turn rancid. Since the vitamins are identical, no one can tell them apart, neither in a test tube nor in an animal. The Health Food Industry designs its advertisements to make you feel vulnerable plus inadequate so you have a need to play it safe and purchase the magical nutrient. How far have we come since Ponce de Leon marched through Florida seeking the "Fountain of Youth?"

The following information on selected vitamins is provided because there is currently special interest in these nutrients. For more in depth information on the vitamins I have omitted, visit your local bookstore, public library, or Internet and refer to the most current texts.

VITAMIN C (Ascorbic acid)

Vitamin C is needed daily in the diet because our bodies cannot manufacture or store it. An adequate supply of Vitamin C prevents scurvy. Scurvy is a disease found in persons with little or no Vitamin C intake over a prolonged period. In scurvy there is bruising, infected gums with loose teeth, bleeding into the joints and muscles of the legs and arms. Finally, if not corrected, jaundice develops, edema (swelling), fever, convulsions, and finally death. This is the classic description of scurvy, and in all my years of practice, I have never seen a case in a child. So please do not think your bruises are due to Vitamin C deficiency.

Cigarette smoking and birth control pills increase the need for Vitamin C. No case has yet been reported of any individual who ate one fruit or vegetable daily and developed scurvy because of smoking.

Megadoses of Vitamin C have been used to treat viral illnesses such as the common cold, hepatitis, influenza, infectious mononucleosis, and pneumonia. The most common side effects of such treatment have been stomach and intestinal upset, diarrhea, abdominal cramping, and flatulence. Lowering the dose of Vitamin C usually eliminates these symptoms. The proponents of this type of vitamin therapy suggest that the dose should be increased to the amount needed to produce these symptoms, then the dose should be lowered slightly. Although there is no strong evidence that Vitamin C prevents the "common cold," there is some evidence that it may decrease the symptoms and shorten the duration of the illness. Many of my patients take Vitamin C supplements and I see as many of these patients as I see who do not take Vitamin C. This, of course, is a non-controlled observation!

Of greater importance is the value of Vitamin C in preventing the conversion of dietary nitrates into a potent carcinogen, nitrosamine. Vitamin C taken daily as a supplement, or even better, daily consumption of foods high in Vitamin C, could decrease the risk of intestinal cancer by preventing nitrosamine formation. Vitamin C also blocks the bacteria Helicobacter pylori, a major cause of stomach ulcer and, possibly, stomach cancer. Citrus fruits, strawberries, melons, tomatoes, broccoli, spinach, potatoes, and green and red peppers are all good sources of Vitamin C, as are a number of tropical fruits, such as kiwi and papaya.

At this time there is a flurry of interest in Vitamin C by eye specialists because, according to animal studies, high levels of Vitamin C in the eye appear to protect against the cataract-inducing effects of ultraviolet radiation from the sun. Prolonged exposure to ultraviolet light is believed to contribute to cataract formation. Middle-aged people who took Vitamin C supplements for many years seem to have lowered their risk of cataracts by as much as 80%. These studies need to be repeated and replicated before accepting them as valid.[67]

Fortunately, most of the warnings about possible toxicity of Vitamin C when it is used as a drug are exaggerated. Compared with the drugs we use daily in medical practice, "over the counter" Vitamin C is a remarkably safe substance.

The story behind discovering the cause of scurvy is fascinating. During the 18th and 19th century, Great Britain needed a large navy to protect and service its colonial-based economy. Scurvy became prevalent when sailors began to spend months at sea without fresh fruit or vegetables. It was of economic importance for Britain to find out what caused scurvy. In 1795, lime juice was given to all British sailors on the recommendation of the Scottish physician, James Lund, who knew that the Dutch had given citrus fruit to its sailors for several hundred years. Gradually, scurvy began to disappear from British sailing ships. That is why British sailors became known as "Limeys."

When I was a student I was told by one of my professors that the American naval medical community refused to believe the claim that limes prevented scurvy. To test the theory, so the story goes, Florida key limes where collected and given to American sailors who were at sea for months. Key limes did not protect the American sailors from scurvy, therefore the theory was rejected. We now know that Florida key limes are the only citrus not to contain Vitamin C! It took many more years before citrus fruit was introduced to the American navy

VITAMIN A (Retinol or beta-carotene)

As a child, the worst part of my day was preparing for bed. That was the time for Cod Liver Oil. In those years, water soluble vitamins did not exist. Thus the natural Vitamin A was given to most children of my generation. The oil was so horrific, I can still taste and smell those vitamin drops. This experience must have been shared by other children because one major complication of taking cod liver oil was pneumonia. Small amounts of the oil would get into the lungs after a struggling child had a gagging or choking spell. This fat soluble vitamin, offered in its natural state, was so irritating to lung tissue that a severe chemical pneumonia developed when the vitamin drops were not totally swallowed but accidentally went down "the wrong tube." Fortunately, we now have a water soluble form and that's what is in children's poly-vitamin drops.

Vitamin A is found in animal products like liver oils, liver, and egg yolk. Retinol is another name for it because it is needed for proper vision. Beta carotene is a provitamin that the body can convert to Vitamin A in the liver. A provitamin, or precursor, is a substance the body can make into a vitamin. It is the carotene that makes vegetables yellow. It is also in green vegetables, but the dark green chlorophyll color conceals it. About 90% of the storable Vitamin A is in the liver.

People with diabetes, low thyroid hormone, and those who use a lot of polyunsaturated fatty acids without antioxidants (Vitamin E) have a decreased ability to convert beta-carotene to Vitamin A. One result of too much carotene in the blood is the formation of a yellow-orange skin color which may be seen in those with untreated diabetes or thyroid disease.

This vitamin is needed to provide normal vision in dim light, bone and tooth enamel growth, and wound healing. It also promotes healthy skin and mucous membranes (the linings of organs, such as the lungs, bladder, stomach, and intestines). Vitamin A improves antibody response and other immune processes to help fight off infection and cancer cells.

Because of all the beneficial effects of Vitamin A, there has been overuse of this vitamin to prevent infection, to improve eyesight, and decrease acne as complications of the "if a little works, more must be better" theory. Side effects of hypervitaminosis A may be encountered, such as terrible headache due to brain swelling, bone and joint pain, hair loss, itching, dry skin, tender bones, weakness, fatigue, and most disastrous, birth defects. Therefore, be sure to remain within the RDA for Vitamin A.[68]

Too much beta-carotene can lead to orange-yellow colored skin which was epidemic in the 1970's when drinking lots of carrot juice was the fad. Fortunately, "carotenosis," as it is called, is of no real consequence and will clear when there is a reduction in carotene intake. Beta carotene, one of more than 40 carotenoids found in food, is one of the most potent antioxidants. The carotenoids are believed to work in concert with other antioxidants. Although beta carotene vitamin pills are popular, they have not been shown to reduce the risk of cancer or heart disease. This is disappointing news, but no surprise since vegetables and fruits contain so many different chemicals in various combination. Our basic understanding of how foods protect us from cancer and heart disease is fragmentary. You would never guess how little we know by reading the exaggerated claims on products sold in gyms and "health food" stores. There will always be someone trying to sell you food supplements of dubious value in this multi-billion dollar market. Below is a table highlighting good sources of four of the over 40 known carotenoids. This underscores what people are missing when they rely on supplements alone. Get your carotene the old fashioned way. Eat carrots, broccoli, squash, spinach, and green leafy vegetables, cantaloupe and other deep yellow, orange fruit. The deeper the color, the higher the carotenoid content.

SOURCES OF COMMON CAROTENOIDS

	BETA-CAROTENE (MICROGRAMS)	LUTEIN & ZEAXANTHIN (MICROGRAMS)	LYCOPENE (MICROGRAMS)
1/2 cup cooked broccoli	1,014	1,404	0
1/2 cup Brussels sprouts	374	1,014	0
1 medium raw carrot	5,688	187	0
1/2 pink grapefruit	1,611	0	4,135
1/2 cup cooked kale	3,055	14,235	0
1 medium peach	86	12	0
1 cup raw spinach	2,296	5,712	0
1 medium tomato	640	123	3,813
3/4 cup tomato juice	1,638	0	15,616

VITAMIN E (Tocopherol)

Vitamin E is another favorite nutrient surrounded with a magical aura. It has been promoted as a substance that increases sexual prowess, fertility, and protects against heart attacks. It is also falsely claimed that Vitamin E applied to a healing wound will diminish the scar.[69]

Pure Vitamin E was first isolated from wheat germ oil in 1936. Although alpha tocopherol is the active compound most often designated as Vitamin E, there are seven other naturally occurring tocopherols. These are designated as (d & l forms) of alpha, beta, gamma, delta, zeta, epsilon, eta, and 8-methyl-tocotrienol and their biological activity varies greatly.

Vitamin E functions as an antioxidant and helps protect polyunsaturated fatty acids in cell membranes and elsewhere in the body. Outside the body it prevents rancidity of oil. Because Vitamin E prevents a process called peroxidation within cells, it was hoped that megadoses of it would protect cells against the aging process and therefore prolong youth and prevent heart attacks. Clinical trials have not provided evidence that routine use of Vitamin E supplements prevents cardiovascular disease or reduces its morbidity (illness) and mortality. Further research is needed to determine whether supplemental Vitamin E has any protective value against coronary heart disease.

Because Vitamin E protects cell constituents from the damaging effects of free radicals that, if unchecked, might contribute to cancer development, it was hoped that Vitamin E would protect against the formation of carcinogenic nitrosamines formed in the stomach from nitrites in foods and enhance the immune system. Unfortunately, human trials and surveys that have attempted to associate Vitamin E intake with cancer incidence have found that Vitamin E is not beneficial in most cases.

Other studies have shown that Vitamin E intake or supplementation did not reduce the risk of prostate cancer.[70]

Very preliminary studies suggesting that Vitamin E may delay the onset of Alzheimer's disease also proved useless.[71]

Meanwhile, the message is to eat foods containing the more complete form of Vitamin E. Fruits and vegetables are the best source of antioxidants because they also provide thousands of phytochemicals that enhance the effects of antioxidants. Rich natural sources of Vitamin E are whole grains, breads and cereals, soybeans, wheat germ oil, safflower oil, lettuce, and most green leafy vegetables.

Laboratory rat experiments demonstrated a heightened sexual potency from Vitamin E, but unfortunately, in humans large doses reduced sexual organ function.[72]

Vitamin E deficiency occurs rarely and produces few symptoms, while excesses can cause headaches, tiredness, giddiness, inflammation of the mouth, chapped lips, muscle weakness, low blood sugar, and a tendency to bleed. By antagonizing the action of Vitamin A, large doses of Vitamin E can also cause blurred vision.

Some of the worst rashes I've seen came from Vitamin E oil repeatedly rubbed on scars. The oil is a potent skin sensitizer. Why then do people use Vitamin E on scars and claim benefits? The answer is relatively simple. There's nothing that heals better than a newly healing scar! In addition, any oil is soothing. Yet most experiments show that anything placed on or in a wound slows healing. My advice is to use a pure vegetable oil if you enjoy the soothing effect, but avoid Vaseline and vitamin oils unless you wish to invite red, bumpy, and irritated skin.

VITAMIN D (Calciferol)

SAFE GUIDELINES FOR VITAMIN D SUPPLEMENTATION

AGE	RDA (IU)	UPPER LEVEL (IU)
1 to 3 years	600	2,500
4 to 8 years	600	3,000
9 to 70 years	600	4,000
71 and older	800	4,000

As discussed earlier, Vitamin D is the "sunshine" vitamin. Because Vitamin D is needed for the normal calcification of bone and teeth, it is very important for the healthy development of a child. Vitamin D is actually more like a hormone than a vitamin. It is produced in the skin and released into the blood to affect bone and other tissues. If the intake of Vitamin D is low or if the child has inadequate sun exposure, even with sufficient dietary calcium and phosphorous, a child or adult will have poor calcification of bone. Menopausal women who take calcium supplements without Vitamin D3 will not receive optimal benefits from taking calcium. Because most milk is fortified with Vitamin D, deficiency of this vitamin in children is seldom a problem in this country. Now with sunscreen use, fewer children playing outdoors in the sun, and less milk drinking amongst teenagers, we are finding more mild to moderate Vitamin D deficiency.

There is evidence from research done on cultured cells (cells isolated from the body and grown in special solutions of nutrients) and in animals with severe Vitamin D deficiency, that Vitamin D (calciferol) is important for activating the immune system. Many scientists believe this discovery provides much needed information about the immune system and it is believed that Vitamin D is an immune modulator. The Health Food Industry is now making wild claims from this basic research, including Vitamin D's ability to stop or control the common cold. Unfortunately, scientific studies sadly found Vitamin D to be as helpful against the common cold as a placebo. There are small studies of high dose Vitamin D supplementation suggesting it helps to lessen the effect of the "common cold."[73]

You should consider supplementing your diet with it if you have tested low in Vitamin D. Taking a daily D3 fish oil supplement or consuming more fatty fish such as salmon, might be suggested by your physician or healthcare provider. In addition, low blood levels of Vitamin D may contribute to the development of peripheral arterial disease. This is a condition of the blood vessels that leads to narrowing and hardening of the arteries that supply the leg and feet. The narrowing of the blood vessels leads to decreased blood flow and causes recurrent leg and calf pain and cramping.

Overweight children 6–18 years old are often found to be Vitamin D deficient. It is not clear whether it is because they spend too much time indoors in front of the TV and computer screen and out of the sun or because their diet is heavy in calories and not heavy in nutrients. The rates of Vitamin D deficiency were higher in Latinos and African-Americans. The particularly high prevalence in severely obese and minority children suggests that targeted screening and treatment guidance is needed.[74]

Vitamin D deficiency is also linked to a variety of chronic conditions, such as:

- High blood pressure
- Type 1 diabetes
- Multiple sclerosis
- Cognitive function
- Depression
- Autoimmune disease

Randomized trials are underway to shed more light on Vitamin D, but results won't be forthcoming for another couple of years. In the meantime, there is concern that Vitamin D deficiency and inadequacy may have been overestimated. The present advice is to keep supplementation within the safe guidelines listed above.

FOLIC ACID (Folate)

Folic acid deficiency may be one of the most common vitamin deficiencies in this country. The word comes from the Latin *folium,* which means "foliage," because it is found in leafy vegetables such as spinach, kale, broccoli, asparagus, chard, sprouts, and other "greens." Folic acid (folate) is available from fresh, unprocessed foods. Many fruits contain folic acid, such as oranges, cantaloupe, pineapple, banana, and many berries, including strawberries, loganberries, and boysenberries. Because so many parents and children live on a diet high in processed foods, they are at risk for folic acid deficiency.

Folic acid (folate) is needed to make DNA, and DNA is needed for cell growth and division. When the body is actively producing cells, as in early pregnancy, there is a tremendous need for extra folate. Since folate, a water soluble B-complex vitamin, is not stored well in the body, humans must consume a constant supply through foods or supplements. If deficiency is present during pregnancy, cell division of the fetus stops, and if this is at a critical time in the development of a fetus (unborn infant), organ formation may be incomplete. Such deformities (called neural tube defects) can result in spina bifida, in which the spinal cord resides outside the spinal column. Defects of the face, including cleft lip and palate, may also occur.[75]

Children with neural tube defects are more likely to have a variant gene that controls the conversion of the amino acid homocysteine to methionine. This mutation may interfere with an intermediate step in the conversion, preventing the overall process from occurring. Researchers have speculated that too much homocysteine prevents the closure of the neural tube, leading to these defects. If the mother consumes adequate amounts of folic acid prior to conception, the conversion of homocysteine to methionine may still proceed, regardless of the child's genetics, and the neural tube may close.[76]

Since these problems occur early in pregnancy, it is especially important for all girls and women of childbearing age to consume a diet high in folate. I recommend that anyone of childbearing age take at least a 0.8 mgs supplement daily. Beginning folate after the critical first few weeks of pregnancy will be too late to correct or prevent the possible damage. When you consider that most women are not even aware of being pregnant until they miss a period, you can see how important it is to develop good dietary habits early. A diet rich in complex carbohydrates, in the form of daily fresh vegetables and fruits is needed if you are to have healthy, normal children. As a public health matter in the United States, flour and breads have been fortified with folic acid for the past few years. Already, the incidence of neural tube defects has decreased.

MINERALS

There are a number of definitions of the word "mineral." In order to understand what mineral means in nutrition, a quick review of some basic chemistry is necessary. Remember that all matter is composed of atoms. There are different types of atoms, such as oxygen, iron, and zinc atoms. These atoms are the basic building blocks of matter. Different types of atoms can combine to form chemical compounds. For example, the atoms hydrogen and oxygen are combined to form the chemical compound water.

Nutritionists use the term "mineral" to refer to the various types of atoms needed by the body. A mineral is an atom or an "element" (not a compound like a vitamin) obtained from food, which is essential to health and is needed in small quantities, sometimes in tiny amounts called "trace elements." Ordinarily, minerals are not eaten in pure form but actually are obtained as part of various compounds in our foods. The body can separate minerals from the food compound in which they are found.

Sodium, calcium, magnesium, and phosphorous are examples of minerals or elements needed by the body, while the minerals, copper, zinc, iron, and iodine are examples of trace elements.

There are 15 major elements of nutritional importance and six are required in relatively large amounts. These include calcium, phosphorous, magnesium, potassium, chloride, and sodium. The remaining nine are essential trace elements: iron, zinc, iodine, manganese, selenium, copper, fluoride, chromium, and molybdenum. These "trace" elements have specific metabolic roles in enzyme systems. Enzymes, as you may recall, are large protein molecules. Most metabolic processes of the body depend on the action of these enzymes.

Not all the minerals listed above will be discussed here. Sodium has already been discussed. Additional information on calcium and iron is included here, but more information is also provided since these minerals are so important to normal growth and development.

CALCIUM

Calcium is the most abundant element or mineral in the body. Not only is it important for our skeleton and bones, but also for nerve conduction, blood clotting, skeletal and heart muscle contraction, and many other metabolic processes. Calcium metabolism is complicated and is just beginning to be understood. The amount of calcium consumed is only one part of a chemical chain of events which include Vitamin D, parathyroid hormones, intestinal absorption, bone mobilization and deposition, urinary excretion, magnesium, phosphates, dietary protein, gravity or weight bearing exercise, and other unknown factors.

Concerns about calcium absorption have arisen in regards to a diet high in phosphorous. This has been of some concern to nutritionists because the consumption of high phosphate foods can decrease absorption. Soft drinks, food additives, and meats are high in phosphates. The possible adverse effects of a continual high phosphate (and high protein) intake on calcium and bone loss should not be taken lightly. A high salt diet also contributes heavily to calcium loss. A diet high in convenience foods such as canned or dehydrated soups, or ready to eat frozen dinners provides an excessive salt, or more correctly, sodium, load to children and adults even if the saltshaker is never used. These long-term effects may be of greater consequence than a low calcium diet.

The need for calcium varies in our life cycle. Needs increase during times of rapid growth of skeleton and muscles, such as pregnancy, lactation, infancy, and especially during adolescence. Not enough calcium in the diet is common in teenage girls on a high soda, candy bar, or "sports bar" diet, but in this group there are multiple nutritional factors that need attention and a "calcium supplement" is only a small part of the answer. An unbalanced diet that has excessive sodium, phosphorous, protein, and insufficient Vitamin D (plus little weight bearing exercise) is a major contributor to calcium deficiency and osteoporosis later in life.

Children and young adults who are bedridden begin to lose calcium and continue to do so until exercise and walking are resumed. Although calcium from dairy products is more completely absorbed, supplementary calcium with Vitamin D may be substituted in those who are unable to tolerate milk. If you take calcium supplements, take them at night because it helps reduce calcium loss into the urine which occurs during sleep, but beware of taking too high a dose of calcium because the excessive amount may help form kidney stones or cause other toxic problems. It is safest to first consult a physician before taking calcium supplements. It is best to avoid supplementation if your dietary calcium is what the RDA suggests. Another piece of sound advice is to cut down on salt, soda (phosphates), and excessive protein because they can remove calcium from the body and counteract the effect of any calcium supplement.

Women who cut the amount of salt in half, from the average of 3,450 mg (about 20 times the amount the adult body needs!) to 1,725 mg of sodium, protect their bones as though a 900mg calcium supplement had been taken. When you consider that one in two women over the age of 50 will fracture a bone due to osteoporosis (a brittle bone condition), you can appreciate how much a high salt diet promotes this condition. A cup of broth, V-8 juice, some cheese, and a salad with anchovies and olives contain enough salt to bump you into calcium-losing mode (and the Margarita or Bloody Mary!)

You may have read that phytates and oxalates in green vegetables make calcium less bioavailable, and this may be true. But as a practical consideration, this is rarely an important problem, given the usual list of calcium rich foods. There is little difference in calcium absorption among sources of calcium as long as supplements are taken with food. If taken on an empty stomach, calcium citrate seems to be absorbed best. Calcium carbonate, although the least expensive, should be taken with food for maximum absorption.

Cheese provides substantial nourishment at the expense of over 50% of calories from fat, most of which is saturated, as well as an enormous salt content. Vegetarians who avoid red meat often unwittingly substitute a large amount of cheese daily. Nutritionally speaking, cream cheese is considered a fat (like butter) and should not be classified with milk, yogurt, and other cheeses. To get the same amount of calcium found in an 8 oz glass of milk, you'd need to eat 13 oz (more than a cup and a half) of regular cream cheese! Do not over-consume cheese or dairy products.

RECOMMENDED DAILY ALLOWANCE FOR CALCIUM

Infants
0 to 6 months	210 mg
7 months to one year	270 mg

Children
1 to 3	700 mg
4 to 8	1000 mg

Women
9 to 18	1300 mg
19 to 50	1000 mg
Over 51	1200 mg
Pregnancy and Lactation	1200 mg
Under 19	1300 mg
Over 19	1000 mg

Men
9 to 18	1300 mg
19 to 50	1000 mg
Over 51	1200 mg

Interpreting labels can be difficult, especially when it comes to understanding mineral needs. The above RDA for calcium is expressed in milligrams of "elemental" calcium. The elemental calcium is the same as usable calcium. For example, if a calcium supplement lists the contents as "calcium citrate = 950 mg" look carefully at the label to see how many milligrams of "calcium" or "elemental" calcium are in the product. If the label says, Calcium (elemental) = 200 mg, that is the amount of calcium the supplement provides. This is true of all minerals. It is the "elemental" iron or "elemental" zinc that is usable.

POTASSIUM

Potassium is an important nutrient found predominantly inside cells. This element, along with sodium, is necessary for electrical impulses to travel along cell membranes. Electrical impulses in body cells are affected by too little or too much potassium. Low potassium causes muscle weakness and heart disturbances while a higher blood potassium could be toxic to the heart. Potassium helps lower blood pressure. A higher potassium, lower sodium diet is helpful in the control and prevention of hypertension. Although most Americans consume excessive sodium, the typical diet is low in potassium. Adults require about 3000 mg of dietary potassium daily. While half a cantaloupe contains 1000 mgs of potassium, and some fruit juices are excellent sources, many children, adolescents and adults consume drinks such as Kool Aid (containing only I mg of potassium), cola drinks (7 mg of potassium), coffee (40 mg of potassium), or beer (36 mg of potassium) instead. Simultaneously, the hundred of milligrams of sodium contained in these drinks drives potassium out of balance. This combination of excess sodium and insufficient potassium contributes to the development of hypertension.

Hypertensive people who take diuretics, lose potassium in their urine along with the sodium. Fatigue is the most common symptom of chronic potassium deficiency. The resulting muscle weakness and fatigue may be gradual and the extent of weakness not fully appreciated until the problem has been corrected.

In childhood, the major causes of potassium deficiency are related to diarrhea and hormonal imbalances. Because potassium regulates heartbeat, adolescents and young adults on a prolonged weight losing diet who consume exclusively a low potassium "liquid protein diet" or those with anorexia nervosa can have a very low heart rate and become gravely ill. Maintaining consistent levels of potassium in the blood and cells is vital to body function.

Potassium is found in a large range of foods, especially oranges, bananas, potatoes (with skin), apricots, prunes, tomatoes, whole grains, legumes, meats, and fish.

MAGNESIUM

Magnesium is an important mineral in human nutrition and shares many of the attributes of calcium. Its distribution in the body is much the same as potassium. Magnesium, calcium, and potassium control the body fluid and keep it from becoming too alkaline or acidic. Magnesium is an integral part of bone crystal, and it activates enzymes for hundreds of reactions including those that involve the expenditure of energy. It is a component of chlorophyll and is also found in animal protein. Good sources of magnesium can be found in whole grains, legumes, dark leafy greens, vegetables, baked potatoes, beans, bananas, apricots, tuna, and salmon.

Because it is found in so many foods and is abundant in nature, magnesium deficiency is extremely rare in healthy people. Deficiencies are mostly seen in persons with alcoholism, persons with diabetes, kidney diseases, and from certain medications such as Nexium. Average consumption from our food is around 300 mg a day.[77]

Young, weight-conscious women appear more susceptible to magnesium deficiency. This may be explained by the common use of diuretics, known to cause deficiency. Liquid protein diets are also associated with magnesium deficiency, as well as a type of potassium deficiency that is difficult to correct.

Grand mal seizures, muscular weakness, heart muscle damage, and heart irregularities are some of the more severe consequences of magnesium deficiency.

Chronic users of PPIs (protein pump inhibitors) such as Nexium or Omeprazole, drugs used to treat acid reflux, may become magnesium depleted and should have a blood test to check their blood level.

CHLORINE

Chlorine is extremely important in electrolyte balance and as its salt, chloride, is a necessary component of gastric juice. Sodium chloride, table salt, is the main provider of chloride in the body. Chloride also aids in the conservation of potassium and while dietary deficiencies are rare, it can be caused by chronic vomiting in childhood and by the overuse of diuretic drugs in adults.

Many years ago, a soybean-based infant formula was removed from the market after it was discovered to contain excessively low amounts of chloride. Some infants consuming this product early in infancy, when no other foods were offered, developed symptoms ranging from marked irritability to severe growth failure. Catastrophes such as this demonstrate how dangerous it is to rely on a single food to provide all our nutrients and points to the danger of fad diets, such as total milk, fruit, and high protein, or "liquid protein diets."[78]

In the late 1960's, Dr. Joseph M. Price published his hypothesis claiming chlorine to be the major cause of cardiovascular disease. He pointed to chlorination of water supply as the origin of heart attacks. To support his argument, he compared the lack of chlorination of water in China, Japan, and parts of Kenya to places where it was present. His figures pointed to a direct relationship between the amount of chlorine consumed and the rate of heart attacks. Advocates of this hypothesis have prepared graphs of "surveys" to support these contentions as reasonable.[79]

The adage, "figures don't lie, but liars figure," comes to mind when data is presented regardless of the source. In spite of my skepticism, I have been caught many times blindly accepting information on face value because a study was performed by a reputable investigator at a prestigious institution. Careful measurements that are reproducible come slowly and with difficulty, but are extremely important if we are to avoid embracing every wild claim by both charlatan and scientist. The chlorine theory has been studied and despite claims of conspiracy that chlorine is a "sacred cow" of the establishment, there is no valid statistical evidence to support these claims. Careful statistical studies have shown no significant relationship between chlorine intake and heart attack rates.

Our drinking water must be guarded against contamination from industrial waste at all costs, but chlorination of our water supply is not only safe, it protects us from waterborne disease capable of causing severe illness. There is a theoretical risk from drinking chlorinated water. Chlorine is known to react with organic material and other pollutants to form traces of chloroform. Chloroform is a carcinogen, and there has been a study linking the presence of chloroform in the water supply to a slightly higher incidence of certain cancers. According to a February 1998 study published in the medical journal, Epidemiology, from the California Department of Health Services, a contaminant, trihalomethanes (THM)[80] commonly found in chlorinated drinking water may be linked to a higher risk of miscarriage among pregnant women who drink five or more glasses of tap water a day. The study found that those pregnant women in their first trimester were roughly twice as likely to have a miscarriage as women who drank less water or whose water had lower concentrations of the contaminant. Health officials said they were taking the results seriously, but stressed that the findings are not definite and need to be confirmed by further research. There is also an association between THMs and the higher occurrence of "Small For Gestational Age" (SGA) infant births. Some health officials recommended that pregnant women find alternatives to unfiltered tap water, such as bottled water.[81]

Despite the undisputed benefits of chlorination in controlling water-borne infectious diseases, the epidemiologic evidence now available suggests that chlorination disinfection by-products (CBPs) may also play a causal role in human bladder cancer.

Monitoring and controlling levels of CBPs in our water supply is an important public health issue and must not be ignored.

Many people choose bottled water because of a fear of their municipal water supply. The water supply in the United States is probably one of the safest in the world, but to keep it so, constant vigilance and support are needed to safeguard our most precious resource. If you use well water, be sure to have it tested for safety.

The water in Flint, Michigan, that was highly contaminated with lead is an example of how the breakdown of the government surveillance systems can destroy lives.[82]

Think of all of those "throw away" plastic bottles contaminating the oceans and waterways. Non-disposable glass containers filled with CBPs free water and kept in the refrigerator are healthier for the environment as well.

IRON

Iron deficiency is one of the most widespread nutritional deficiency problems still seen in the United States. Although there is much written about other minerals and vitamins allegedly being in short supply in our diet, iron deficiency remains a real problem in infancy, adolescence, and especially in pregnancy.

When one thinks of iron deficiency, anemia is the problem that often comes to mind. But depletion of body stores of iron causes many problems in the body long before anemia or low hemoglobin occurs. By the time anemia is present, many other bodily changes have occurred. Vital metalloenzymes are affected early, producing symptoms of irritability and poor appetite in children. Other behavioral changes such as pica, (eating dirt, soil, paint chips, etc.) and the craving for ice frequently occur. It has been suggested that alcoholism has occasionally resulted from this ice craving since it is socially acceptable for adults to drink ice with alcoholic drinks. Allegedly the iron-deficient compulsive ice eater gets habituated to the alcohol as well. Treatment with oral iron supplements results in the disappearance of the ice craving, poor appetite, and irritability usually within a week or two, and long before the anemia itself is corrected. Chronic fatigue is believed to be a relatively late symptom in iron deficiency, but decreased work performance has been found in people with even mild iron deficiency.

Researchers from Johns Hopkins Medical School reported in the British medical journal Lancet their study in which 700 teenage girls in Baltimore high schools were screened for iron deficiency. Scientists were looking for girls with low iron levels, but not low enough to cause anemia. This study's screening method differed from how most physicians screen for low iron levels. Usually physicians check a simple hemoglobin or hematocrit. If anemia is not found, it is assumed that iron levels are adequate. But anemia reflects only severe iron deficiency. Moderately low iron levels can exist without anemia.

The researchers found 73 girls, roughly 10%, who had low iron levels, but who had not yet developed iron deficiency anemia. These girls were then screened with several standardized tests to measure verbal learning skills and memory. The group of girls were then divided into two groups, making sure that both groups had similar levels of iron deficiency and similar test scores.

Half the girls were then treated with iron pills and the other were given identical placebos containing no iron. After eight weeks, the girls were re-tested. The half that were given iron had higher blood iron levels and higher blood counts. This result was expected, but in addition this group also did significantly better on the verbal learning and memory tests. Eight weeks of iron therapy was effective in improving scores on these important measures of brain function in iron-deficient high school girls.[83]

It is extremely rare for older teenage boys or young adult men to be anemic due to lack of iron. Anemia in adult men should always be thoroughly investigated for its cause. Taking iron tablets could hide and postpone early diagnosis or recognition of blood loss in the stool from colitis, polyps, or intestinal cancer.

Be sure to have all pills or medicines locked up or out of reach of climbing toddlers and young children. Iron poisoning remains one of the more common and often deadly poisonings in children. Poison Centers have become increasingly alarmed about the number of iron poisonings in young children. Iron poisonings kill more children under age six than any other substance and most of these poisonings occur as a result of children accidentally ingesting iron tablets or prenatal vitamins. As few as ten tablets of 325 mg ferrous sulfate can be fatal to a child weighing less than 22 pounds. Treatment of iron poisoning should not be delayed. If your child swallows iron pills, call your doctor and go to the emergency room right away!

Doctors often test for anemia with a simple hemoglobin test. The results might appear normal, and a patient may have no obvious illness, but iron deficiency may still exist. This is especially so during periods of rapid growth as during infancy, adolescence, and throughout the child-bearing period in women. During these times when demand for iron for hemoglobin formation and muscle is increased, additional iron is needed in the diet. Especially at risk are premature infants and children 6 months to 3 years of age. Regular aspirin users are also at high risk for iron deficiency. For these reasons, iron fortification has been promoted by public health-minded nutritionists.

Rather than relying on people to remember to take extra iron every day in pill form, iron has been added to flour and cereal. For those who prefer to get their iron from more natural sources, good ones are whole wheat, fish, poultry (the dark meat has more iron than white meat), figs, dates, beans, asparagus, black strap molasses, oatmeal, enriched bread, dark green vegetables, and extra lean meat. One cup of prune juice supplies 55% of an adult woman's RDA for iron. Cooking in iron pots and pans contributes a great deal of extra iron to the diet. The much fabled spinach, Popeye's ready source, has many milligrams of iron, but in the form of poorly absorbable iron oxalate. Even the iron in egg yolk may not be as absorbable as once thought. Broccoli has significantly more available iron (and calcium). Phosphates, found in sodas, also form compounds with iron which are difficult for the body to absorb.

Some foods decrease iron absorption. Bran and teas containing tannin are two. (Coffee which contains no tannins, depresses absorption, but to a lesser degree.) More than a quart of milk a day also contributes to iron deficiency.

In contrast, other foods increase iron absorption, particularly Vitamin C rich foods. The Vitamin C counteracts the effects of other iron inhibitors.

The Vitamin C changes the poorly absorbable ferric iron found in many foods to the more soluble ferrous form. Vitamin C, however, is not an important enhancer of iron pill absorption since it is already in the ferrous form. This is important to remember, especially for pregnant women, who are often advised to take high doses of iron supplements. Taking a ferrous iron pill before breakfast insures excellent absorption. Small amounts of animal protein such as beef, poultry, or fish added to a meal can increase iron absorption from food fourfold.

Many people wish to take iron supplements because of the fact that the bioavailability of iron in foods varies so greatly. In the ordinary diet 10–20 mg of iron are consumed each day, but less than 10% of this is absorbed. The requirements for iron found in the RDA take into account the low amount of iron actually absorbed from iron pills. I tell my patients that in recommended doses iron is safe, but to be careful not to consume too much iron as a supplement because in large amounts it can be toxic and cause abdominal discomfort. Ferrous sulfate is a good supplement to take if needed, as it is very well absorbed. Some chelated iron compounds which are sold because of its less irritating effect on the gut, are often passed out in the stool without being absorbed.

Infant formulas should have 12–18 mg of iron per quart. Breastfed infants get iron from breast milk in adequate amounts because of its extremely high bioavailability. Fortified infant cereals should not be feared. They are especially nutritious and contain the type of additives that are nutritionally desirable. Premature infants especially, if not breastfed, should be on an iron fortified formula and extra iron daily if recommended by the neonatologist or physician.

Heavy menstrual periods are a frequent contributor to iron deficiency, which is why women after puberty and during childbearing years are frequently iron deficient. It is very popular now for many men and women to totally avoid red meat. Women who avoid red meat are especially vulnerable to iron deficiency without obvious symptoms and might benefit from a small daily iron supplement. It is extremely rare for an adult man to be anemic due to lack of iron. Anemia in adult men should always be thoroughly investigated for its cause. Taking iron tablets could hide and postpone early diagnosis or recognition of blood loss in the stools from colitis, polyps, kidney disease, or intestinal cancer.

RECOMMENDED DAILY ALLOWANCES
FOR ELEMENTAL IRON

Infants

0-6 months	10 mg	
6 months to 3 years	15 mg	

Children	4–10 years	10 mg

Males & Females	11–18 years	18 mg
Males	19 & over	10 mg
Females	19–50 years	18 mg
	51 & over	10 mg

Pregnancy	36 mg
Lactation (breastfeeding mothers)	18 mg

The above RDA for Iron is expressed in milligrams of "elemental" iron. The elemental iron is the same as usable iron. For example, there are 220 mg of ferrous sulfate in one teaspoon of the elixir (liquid form) and this equals 50 mg of elemental iron. The usual tablet of ferrous sulfate is 325 mg, but it delivers 65 mg of elemental iron.

ZINC

In 1963, zinc was first recognized as an essential element for humans. A normal American diet easily supplies the RDA for zinc because most Americans eat animal protein and zinc is found in abundant amounts in all meats. Diets which exclude meat, fish, and other zinc rich foods such as eggs, milk, and whole grains, may produce symptoms of zinc deficiency.

Deficiency is also a potential problem in alcoholics with liver disease, patients with chronic kidney disease, rheumatoid arthritis, inflammatory bowel disease, and malabsorption syndrome (nutrients poorly absorbed from the gut). The rash that is characteristic of zinc deficiency resembles eczema. It occurs on the face, hands, feet, and ano-genital regions. Other signs of zinc deficiency are loss of appetite, loss of taste, and possibly slower wound healing. These symptoms can also appear in individuals following an unusual crash diet.

At the opposite end of the spectrum is zinc toxicity due to zinc overdose. As with zinc deficiency, this is extremely rare, except in cases in which a person has been taking large zinc supplements and has a diet which is already high in zinc. Sometimes zinc poisoning (toxicity) is due to ingesting foods stored in galvanized containers. Water that flows through galvanized pipes does not pose a problem, however. Symptoms of zinc toxicity are stomach upset, nausea, vomiting, bleeding in the stomach, and anemia secondary to this blood loss. Long-term zinc overdose can also interfere with resistance to infection.

Zinc deficiency in humans was first reported in the early 1960s in very short individuals found to be on a diet low in meat and fish, but very high in bread made from grains high in phytates. Phytates are known to bind zinc and thus inhibit its uptake in the body. Upon treatment with supplemental zinc these patients showed a striking response in growth and development of their secondary sex characteristics. Immediate responses to zinc supplementation in deficient persons include personality changes, clearing of skin lesions as well as increased body growth, particularly in infants. Children with zinc deficiency are extremely irritable and difficult to manage. The first response to zinc supplementation in deficient young children is that they become more placid, usually within 24 hours after the first treatment.

Recently, intriguing studies have suggested that zinc lozenges, when started within 24 hours of symptoms, may be effective in reducing the symptoms and duration of the common cold by up to 42%.[84] A study showed that if zinc lozenges were started with 24 hours of onset of cold symptoms, and administered no less than two hours apart (up to eight lozenges per day) cold symptoms lasted only 4.3 versus the 9.2 days found in a matched placebo group. Researchers aren't sure how zinc affects the common cold but they do know that in a test tube, zinc stops many cold viruses from multiplying. To date, more than 300 zinc-dependent enzymes have been identified, thus promoting multiple theories on how zinc might work in preventing the common cold. It may induce the production of interferon or the effect may be due in part to correction of subclinical zinc deficiency in selected persons. There is no shortage of theories! Whatever the mechanism, these recent studies raise the intriguing possibility that zinc may be effective in reducing the duration and severity of the common cold. Unfortunately, zinc is not always well tolerated. Ninety percent of those taking zinc lozenges (23 mg of elemental zinc usually as zinc gluconate) reported mild to moderate side effects such as nausea and bad taste.[85]

Carefully conducted studies are needed before this therapy can be recommended, especially to children. If zinc becomes a widely used remedy against the common cold, long-term surveillance will be necessary to verify its safety. Much of the commercial hype about zinc's ability to prevent or modify the common cold is overstated.

THE RECOMMENDED DIETARY ALLOWANCE FOR ZINC RDA

Infants 0–12 months	5 mg
Children 1–10 years old	10 mg
Males 11–51+	15 mg
Females 11–51+	12 mg
Pregnancy	15 mg
Lactation 1st 6 months	19 mg
2nd 6 months	16 mg

FLUORINE (FLUORIDE)

When communities began to add fluoride, a fluorine containing salt, to drinking water in the 1960's, rates of tooth decay fell by 50 to 60 percent. Fluoride strengthens tooth enamel, making it more resistant to acids formed in the mouth by sugar fermenting bacteria. For those children living outside of water districts that fluoridate their water, bottled fluoridated water, fluoride drops or pills are almost as effective as drinking fluoridated water. But even the most motivated parent knows it is difficult to remember to give a child that daily fluoride pill for ten or more years. Parents often are more motivated to give a daily multivitamin to their child, so fluoride is often prescribed combined with a multivitamin and these preparations work as well as if they were given separately.

Fluoride given on an empty stomach is 100% absorbed, but when given with milk or a calcium rich meal, it is incompletely absorbed. Fluoridated toothpaste is very popular and is of value in reducing cavities. Very little toothpaste is needed to brush teeth adequately, and since many young children swallow toothpaste, it is prudent to keep the amount of paste to a small bead. Too much fluoride can cause slight mottling of the tooth enamel. The risk of mottling can be reduced by carefully following the current recommended supplementation dosages by the American Academy of Pediatrics Committee on Nutrition.[86] Fluoride also favors the deposition of calcium, thereby strengthening bones and may help prevent osteoporosis. This has not been substantiated in large studies. The safety and nutrition advantages that result from fluoridation of the water supply have been demonstrated, but there are those who feel our water supply should not be tampered with. Although the argument for "freedom of choice" may be valid, the scare tactics used by anti-fluoridationists are unsupported by reputable studies. The amount added—one part fluoride to one million parts of water—does not cause cancer, nor is fluoridation a foreign plot to weaken our children's bodies, as some claim.

Breast milk, cow milk, prepared infant foods, beverages, and sodas contain virtually no fluoride. Various food snacks have been graded for their cavity-producing capacity. Snack raisins are the worst, followed by cookies, sticky candy bars, doughnuts, and pre-sweetened cereals; then nut butters, chips, and soda pop. While on the subject of tooth decay, I would be remiss not to mention fruit juices. Fruit juice is pure sugar. That's right—natural sugar, but nonetheless sugar. I frequently observe parents giving three bottles of juice a day to their infants and toddlers to use as a pacifier. This means that the child washes his or her teeth with sugar constantly, which leads to "apple juice teeth." It need not be apple juice, it can be any fruit juice or even cow or breast milk (they contain the milk sugar, lactose). In addition to tooth decay, the sugar in fruit juice often is responsible for a poor appetite and results in a very irritable child. Limit juice to once a day and if you must use the "bottle" as a pacifier, fill it with pure water, and not dilute juice.

Supplementation of the diet is no substitute for a wholesome diet. To achieve and maintain healthy teeth and gums throughout life, oral hygiene, optimal nutrition, and avoidance of sticky snacks are critical.

FLUORIDE SUPPLEMENTATION SCHEDULE

- No supplementation for water containing over 0.6 ppm fluoride.
- No supplementation for infants under six months of age.
- No supplementation for children under three years of age where fluoride level is over 0.3 ppm.

Discuss with your dentist whether there is a need to supplement with fluoride or if periodic dental application is sufficient, because recommendations may change with new information.

SELENIUM

Recent studies suggest that selenium might be involved in a variety of important biological processes, including those of the immune system. Animal studies have demonstrated that selenium offers some protection against environmental carcinogens. Selenium is one of a group of minerals including zinc, copper, iron, and manganese which help neutralize free radicals. That is, they help fight cell damage caused by oxygen derived compounds, and thus may protect against certain cancers. For these reasons, it has been recommended that malnourished people take selenium as a supplement up to a maximum of 50 micrograms a day. However, selenium can also be quite toxic and the range between safe and too much is very narrow.

In the general population, dietary selenium intake varies greatly, depending on the type of food consumed and the geographic location in which these foods are produced. Selenium is not distributed evenly in agricultural lands. As a result, many of our foods are grown in selenium deficient soils. Since selenium is not essential for the growth of grains, fertilizers usually do not contain selenium. In the United States and Canada it has been reported that the more selenium found in the soil and farm crops, the lower the human cancer rate in those areas.

Keshan disease is a potentially fatal heart muscle and muscle weakness disease found in young children deficient in selenium. It is seen in China where selenium is deficient in the soil. It is occasionally seen in premature infants kept on intravenous fluids for weeks when the nutrient fluid has no added selenium. Selenium supplementation programs in China have eradicated this widespread problem.

Fortunately, seafood, especially oysters, halibut, swordfish, salmon, and tuna, is rich in selenium and is an excellent low fat source of protein as well. Other foods rich in selenium include yeast, asparagus, garlic, whole grains, and cashews. Although kelp is rich in selenium, many other toxic metals such as arsenic and mercury may also be present.

COPPER

Copper is an essential nutrient which the body stores in the liver. It is crucial to respiration, hemoglobin synthesis, bone and connective tissue growth, and normal function of the central nervous system. There are several extremely rare causes of copper deficiency at birth that have to do with genetic inborn errors of metabolism (Wilson's disease, Menke's disease). Copper deficiency due to inadequate intake of this mineral is primarily seen in patients fed for long periods on intravenous fluid deficient in this mineral. An early feature of nutritional copper deficiency is anemia unresponsive to iron therapy. Large quantities of supplemental zinc can also impair copper absorption. On a practical level, copper deficiency should not be a concern to parents.

Good dietary sources of copper are shellfish, (especially oysters), beans, nuts, whole grains, and potatoes.

IODINE

Iodine is needed for normal cell metabolism and for the thyroid gland to make thyroid hormones. Insufficient intake of this trace element can lead to a goiter due to enlargement of the thyroid gland. Goiters were once common in parts of the world, called "goiter belts," where the soil was deficient in iodine. In the United States, the goiter belt included the Great Lakes region and the Plains states. In the 1930s, about 40% of the people in Michigan had a goiter due mainly to iodine deficiency. As a public health measure, iodized salt was introduced, and although we still see goiters in America, they are rarely due to iodine deficiency.

Cretinism, a form of mental retardation, is found in infants born with little or no thyroid hormone and was once commonly caused by iodine deficiency. The mental retardation of cretinism can be prevented by giving these infants thyroid hormone immediately after birth. Most newborns in the United States are screened by a blood test to help obtain an early diagnosis of this preventable disaster.

The best sources of iodine are iodized salt, seafood, and dairy products and crops grown from iodine rich areas. It is extremely unlikely that iodine deficiency would occur in children or adults on a low salt diet, since only minuscule amounts are needed—micrograms—and therefore supplementation is rarely needed. Most multivitamin-mineral supplements contain 150 mcg.

L-carnitine is a nutrient made within our body from two amino acids, lysine and methionine. This compound is found in high concentration in beef, pork, and bacon. Intestinal bacteria, via a series of steps, has been shown to convert l-carnitine to a substance trimethylamine-N-oxide or better known as TMAO. This compound has recently been demonstrated to accelerate atherosclerosis in mice. This may be an explanation of why there is a link between high levels of red meat consumption and cardiovascular risk.[87] Teens who take carnitine as a dietary supplement should be made aware of this connection. This is one more reason to be wary of dietary supplements.

PRODUCT/100 grams   CARNITINE

Beef steak	95 mg
Ground beef	94 mg
Pork	27.7 mg
Bacon	23.3 mg
Tempeh	19.5 mg
Cod fish	5.6 mg
Chicken breast	3.9 mg
American cheese	3.7 mg
Cottage cheese	1.1 mg

CHAPTER 18

The New Nutrition Facts Label: What's in It for You?[88]

The US Food and Drug Administration (FDA) has updated the nutrition facts label on packaged foods and drinks.

#1 The serving size now appears in larger, bold font and some serving sizes have been updated. This is more realistic and reflects what people typically eat.

#2 Calories are now displayed in larger, bolder font.

#3 Daily Value has been updated.

#4 Added sugars, Vitamin D, and potassium are now listed.

Manufacturers must declare the amount in addition to percent Daily Value for vitamins and minerals.

Vitamin A and C are no longer required on the label since deficiencies of these vitamins are rare today.

Another important addition to the label is the added sugars such as sucrose, table sugar, sugars from syrups and honey, and sugars from concentrated fruit or vegetable juices.

Vitamin D and potassium are now listed. Potassium can reduce the risk of high blood pressure.

For your information, I have included a generic version of a nutrition facts label on the following page.

Serving Size ➡️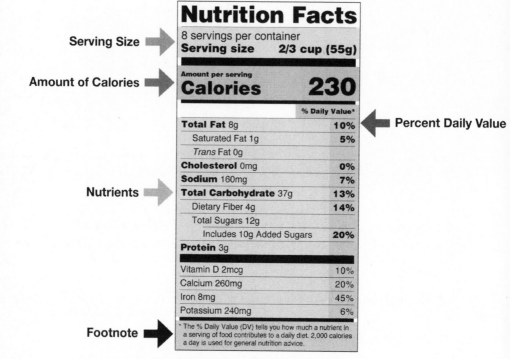

Amount of Calories ➡️

Nutrients ➡️

Footnote ➡️

⬅️ Percent Daily Value

Nutrition Facts

8 servings per container
Serving size   2/3 cup (55g)

Amount per serving
Calories   230

	% Daily Value*
Total Fat 8g	**10%**
Saturated Fat 1g	**5%**
Trans Fat 0g	
Cholesterol 0mg	**0%**
Sodium 160mg	**7%**
Total Carbohydrate 37g	**13%**
Dietary Fiber 4g	**14%**
Total Sugars 12g	
Includes 10g Added Sugars	**20%**
Protein 3g	
Vitamin D 2mcg	10%
Calcium 260mg	20%
Iron 8mg	45%
Potassium 240mg	6%

* The % Daily Value (DV) tells you how much a nutrient in
a serving of food contributes to a daily diet. 2,000 calories
a day is used for general nutrition advice.

*(For educational purposes only. These labels do not meet
the labeling requirements described in 21 CFR 101.9.)*

This label is courtesy of the U.S. Food and Drug Administration.
For a free downloadable copy similar to this one, see
https://www.fda.gov/media/132224/download.

CHAPTER 19

Definitions

Low in saturated fat: No more than one gram of saturated fat per individual serving or less than 10% of calories from saturated fat in a meal or main dish.

Light or "Lite": The fat content or calories must be cut in half. The label should tell which one. Light can also mean one half the usual sodium content.

Lean: The USDA defines lean as less than 10 grams of fat in the meal; less than 4 grams of saturated fat, and less than 95 mg of cholesterol (per 100 grams or 3.5 ounces).

Extra-lean: Less than 5 grams of fat in a meal or main dish; less than 2 grams of saturated fat, and less than 95 mg of cholesterol (per 100 grams or 3.5 ounces).

Cholesterol Free: Less than 2 mg of cholesterol

Good source: Must contain at least 10% of the Daily Value of the nutrient.

High source: Must contain at least 20% of the Daily Value of the nutrient.

"Good source" or "High source" could be used deceptively by suggesting this is a healthy food. For example, if a meal contains a vegetable such as broccoli, the package may claim "Contains broccoli, a good source of folic acid" but have a high salt or sodium content.

Calories: The total calories per serving.

Calorie-free: Fewer than 5 calories per serving

Low Calorie: 40 calories or less per serving (and per 50 grams of food).

Reduced Calories: A product altered to contain 25 percent fewer calories than the comparable food without reduced calories.

Sugar Free: Less than 1/2 gram per serving.

Sodium Free: Less than 5 mg per serving

Low Sodium: Less than 140 mg per serving and per 50 grams of food.

Very Low Sodium: Less than 35 mg per serving and per 50 grams of food.

Sodium, Lite or Light: If the sodium content of a low-calorie, low-fat food has been reduced by half.

Fresh Frozen: freshly frozen, frozen fresh. (A conflict of meanings!)

A Source of: One serving must contain at least 10–19 percent of the adult daily requirement of the named nutrient.

Reduced or Less: Contains at least 25 percent less of the named substance than the food usually contains.

Ingredients: Ingredients are listed by weight, from the most to the least. If corn syrup, molasses, sugar, maltose, fructose are high on the list, the food probably is loaded with simple sugars. When oil, butter, hydrogenated fats or oils, cheese, or lard are represented high on the list, the food may have excessive amounts of saturated fats and cholesterol. When the ingredients label says, "May contain one or more of the following: soybean oil and/or palm oil," it means either one may be substituted for the other (usually depending upon which one is less expensive or more available at the moment). Look for the words, salt, sodium, soy sauce, sodium bicarbonate, seaweed, and sea salt as indicators that you are dealing with a high salt food.

The most important thing to remember is that the ingredients are listed in descending order of predominance. The first two or three ingredients are the ones that matter most.

Prevention of Nutritional Losses from Foods[89]

Storing, processing, and cooking of fresh vegetables can cause nutritional losses. As a generalization, minerals, carbohydrates, fats, protein, Vitamin K, and niacin are stable (greater than 85% retention) during processing and storage of foods. The nutrients most affected by cooking at home are the B-complex vitamins and Vitamin C because these vitamins dissolve in water and are usually drained away in the cooking water. Prolonged cooking in too much water as well as cutting vegetables into small pieces before cooking (processing) tends to increase vitamin loss.

A basic rule for maintaining the nutrients is to cook vegetables in water which weighs no more than 1/3 as much as the food. For example, if you were to cook a pound of vegetables you would need only 1/3 of a pound of cooking water. One pound of water is equivalent to one pint, so 1/3 of a pound of water would amount to less than a cup. One pint of water would be 2 cups. If cooking water does not cover the vegetable, steam from the boiling water will still cook it completely.

It is important to limit the cooking water only if it is to be discarded. If it is saved to be eaten in soup, it makes no difference—the vitamins remain. Just as your grandmother said, save the water for the soup!

To further reduce all vitamin losses, cook your food no longer than is necessary to suit your taste. Food should be cooked as soon before serving as possible since the nutritional value of food is highest at that time.

Steaming brings less water into contact with vegetables than boiling. But steam still wets the vegetables and the water drips back into the pan. Steaming and boiling in a small quantity of water are nearly equal in removing vitamins.

Microwaving is a rapid method of cooking and causes minimal vitamin loss!

Storage of cooked vegetables for a day or longer in the refrigerator and then reheated results in losses of Vitamin C between 25 to 50%. Vitamins in foods are also destroyed when stored in the freezer. The colder the refrigerator or freezer, the smaller the loss will be. Concentrated frozen orange juice refrigerated one year loses only 5% of the Vitamin C. As a rule, however, there can be a significant loss of nutritional value when a food is stored longer than a few months in the freezer. Freezing slows destruction of nutrients but does not completely stop the destruction.

Vitamin A is reasonably stable in almost all food products and processes, with a notable exception of dehydrated foods exposed to air. Extended cooking of green, yellow, or red vegetables can lower the Vitamin A by 15–35%, but cooking high fiber foods such as carrots probably increases the absorption of Vitamin A.

Folic acid losses average only 10% during baking while prolonged cooking of meat destroys this B Vitamin.

Vitamin D is sensitive to light and that is why milk should be stored in opaque containers such as cartons rather than clear glass bottles

TIPS TO BOOST VITAMINS AND MINERALS IN YOUR DIET

1. Purchase only the freshest vegetables and fruits because vitamins are lost when produce is wilted, bruised, or old.

2. Darker colored vegetables are generally richer in nutrients. Dark green salad leaves for example, provide more Vitamin A and iron than lighter ones. Orange carrots have more Vitamin A than paler, yellow carrots. Yellow corn is more nutritious than white corn.

3. Pay attention to "sell before" expirations dates on milk and cottage cheese containers. Select the "youngest" product to assure freshest flavor and best maintenance of B Vitamins.

4. Avoid overcooking meat and fish. Medium or medium rare rather than well-done meat or seafood contains more B-1 (thiamine). An exception is hamburger meat. All ground meat should be cooked well done, to kill any contaminating bacteria.

5. Refrigerate leftover vegetables as soon as possible and use them within a day or two.

6. Potatoes, onions, carrots, and sweet potatoes keep best in a cool place (about 50 degrees F).

7.   Ripen tomatoes at room temperature and then refrigerate when ripe. Use as soon as they are ripe because tomatoes lose Vitamin C with aging.

8.   Fresh vegetables should be used soon after purchase. Vitamins and flavor are lost when vegetables are kept too long in the refrigerator.

Vision for the Future:
The Science of Nutrition

I propose several questions that need to be answered:

- What is the best diet?
- What and when should we eat?
- What do we need to eat and how does it affect us?
- How does what we eat promote health across our lifespan?
- How do we improve the use of food as medicine?
- How do we correct minority health and health disparities?
- What role does nutrition play in the microbiome of the gut and its influence on immunity, the brain, and psychological conditions?

To answer these questions we need innovative research and a strategy from the NIH. The National Institute of Health is the branch of our government with the most experience to date for modernizing unbiased nutrition research. We must learn what diets are best for health, disease prevention, and longevity.

Acknowledgments

How shall I feed my child and family?" is on the mind of every parent. I am grateful to the many people who helped me answer this question. My friend, Joan F. Green, deserves special recognition for her critical review of each page of this book and encouraging me to submit, *Feed Your Body Right: from Birth through Adulthood*, for publication. Thanks to my wife, Linda Goldberg, RN OB-GYN Nurse Practitioner for proofreading, making multiple suggestions to improve this book and especially for her patience with me during this time.

HAVE A COMMENT, A QUESTION, OR AN IDEA?

Send us an email!

(Our email address can be found at **sanrafaelpediatrics.com.**)

We respond to all emails!

Endnotes

1. See MedlinePlus, https://medlineplus.gov/druginfo/meds, under "T." Accessed December 15, 2020.

2. For more information on these diseases, see BMJ Journals, Archives of Disease in Childhood, https://adc.bmj.com/. Accessed December 15, 2020.

3. Ibid.

4. For more information about organic farming and Rodale's farm, see Rodale Institute's website, https://rodaleinstitute.org/. Accessed December 15, 2020.

5. Susan C. Schena, "Marin Ranks As Healthiest County In California: Report," Patch.com, Mar 20, 2019. See https://patch.com/california/novato/marin-ranks-healthiest-county-california-report. Accessed December 14, 2020.

6. Wikipedia, "Ketchup as a Vegetable." See https://en.wikipedia.org/wiki/Ketchup_as_a_vegetable#:~:text=After%20President%20Reagan%20re-moved%20the,daily%20nutrients%20in%20school%20lunches. Accessed December 14, 2020.

7. Jillian Kubala, "Hydrogen water: miracle drink of overhyped myth?" Healthline, Jan. 16, 2019. See www.healthline.com/nutrition/hydrogen-water.

8. Mandy Oaklander, "Salt Doesn't Cause High Blood Pressure?" Here's What a New Study Says," *Time* magazine, Sept. 10, 2014. See time.com3313332/salt-and-blood-pressure.

9. Feeding Littles, "What's the Deal with Babies and Salt?" See https://www.feedinglittles.com/blog/whats-the-deal-with-babies-and-salt. Accessed December 14, 2020.

10. *The American Journal of Clinical Nutrition*, Volume 77, Issue 6, June 2003, 1489–497.

11. Ibid.

12. Fiona Godlee, "The Food Industry Fights for Salt," *BMJ*, 1996;312:1239. See https://doi.org/10.1136/bmj.312.7041.1239.

13. Anahad O'Connor, "How the Sugar Industry Shifted Blame to Fat," New York Times, Sept. 12, 2016. See https://www.nytimes.com/2016/09/13/well/eat/how-the-sugar-industry-shifted-blame-to-fat.html.

14. Camila Domonoske, "50 Years Ago, Sugar Industry Quietly Paid Scientists to Point Blame at Fat," NPR's *The Two-Way*, Sept. 13, 2016. See https://www.npr.org/sections/thetwo-way. Accessed December 14, 2020.

15. T. Tanvetyanon and G. Bepler, "Beta-carotene in multivitamins and the possible risk of lung cancer among smokers versus former smokers: a meta-analysis and evaluation of national brands," *Cancer*, Jul. 1, 2008, 13:150–57.

16. "Medical Foods Market to Reach USD 29.54 Billion By 2026 | Reports and Data," Globe Newswire, June 10, 2019. See https://www.globenewswire.com/news-release/2019/06/10/1866412/0/en/Medical-Foods-Market-To-Reach-USD-29-54-Billion-By-2026-Reports-And-Data.html. Accessed December 15, 2020.

17. Mahmoud Rafieian-Kopaei, Mahbubeh Setorki, Monir Doudi, Azar Baradaran, Hamid Nasri, "Atherosclerosis: Process, Indicators, Risk Factors and New Hopes," Int J Prev Med. 2014 Aug; 5(8): 927–946.

18. Ibid.

19. For more information on the Pritkin diet, see the Home Fitness on Top website, https://www.homefitnessontap.com/.

20. Robert C. Atkins, Dr. Atkins New Diet Revolution (New York: Harper, Dec. 2009).

21. Jenna Fletcher, "Keto diet side effects: What to expect," MedicalNewsToday, June 22, 2020. See https://www.medicalnewstoday.com/articles/keto-diet-side-effects.

22. "PREDIMED: Study Retration and Republication," The Nutrition Source, Harvard School of Public Health, June 22, 2018. See https://www.hsph.harvard.edu/nutritionsource/2018/06/22/.

23. Ibid.

24. T. Colin Campbell and Thomas M. Campbell II, *The China Study*, revised edition (Dallas, TX: BenBella, 2016).

25. Joe Conason, "Bill Clinton embraces this vegan diet," AARP, *The Magazine*, August/September 2013.

26. Leonardo Trasande, Rachel M. Shaffer, Sheela Sathyanarayana, and the Council on Environmental Health, "Food Additives and Child Health," *Pediatrics*, August 2018, 142 (2) e20181410; DOI: https://doi.org/10.1542/peds.2018-1408.

27. Luoping Zhang, Lemaan Rana, Rachel M. Shaffer, Emanuela Taioli, and Lianne Sheppard, "Exposure to glyphosate-based herbicides and risk for non-Hodgkin lymphoma: A meta-analysis and supporting evidence," *Science Direct*, See https://www.sciencedirect.com/science/article/abs/pii/S1383574218300887?via%3Dihub. Accessed December 11, 2020.

28. Mike Belliveau, "Letter: (Re)emergence of phthalates in food," Environmental Health News, Dec. 29, 2017. See https://www.ehn.org/phthalates-in-food-2520481250.html.

29. Shaina L. Stacy, George D. Papandonatos, Antonia M. Calafat, Aimin Chen, Kimberly Yolton, Bruce P. Lanphear, and Joseph M. Braun 7, "Early life bisphenol A exposure and neurobehavior at 8 years of age: Identifying windows of heightened vulnerability," National Library of Medicine, PubMed.gov, October 2017, 107:258–65. See https://pubmed.ncbi.nlm.nih.gov/28764921/. Accessed December 14, 2020.

30. Cheryl Erler, DNP, RNA and Julie Novak, DNSc, RN, CPNP, FAANPB, "Bisphenol A Exposure: Human Risk and Health Policy." See https://www.pediatricnursing.org/article/S0882-5963(09)00140-7/fulltext. Accessed December 11, 2020.

31. Nicole Greenfield, "The Pesticide in Your Crisper Drawer," NRDC, May 2, 2017. See https://www.nrdc.org/stories/pesticide-your-crisper-drawer?.

32. Olga V. Naidenko, "Application of the Food Quality Protection Act children's health safety factor in the U.S. EPA pesticide risk assessments," Environmental Health, Feb. 10, 2020. See https://ehjournal.biomedcentral.com/articles/10.1186/s12940-020-0571-6.

33. Nicole Greenfield, "The Pesticide in Your Crisper Drawer," NRDC, May 2, 2017. See https://www.nrdc.org/stories/pesticide-your-crisper-drawer?.

34. Jeff Daniels, "Big battle ahead as California considers banning farm pesticide Trump's EPA supports," NBR.com, July 21, 2017. See https://www.cnbc.com/2017/07/21/california-considers-banning-a-farm-pesticide-trumps-epa-supports.html. Accessed December 14, 2020.

35. Olivia Nugroho, "The Dirty Dozen: Why Organic is Best," Riordan Clinic, https://riordanclinic.org/2017/11/the-dirty-dozen-organic-best/.

36. "7 Tips for Cleaning Fruits, Vegetables," U.S. Food and Drug Administration, June 10, 2018. See https://www.fda.gov/consumers/consumer-updates/7-tips-cleaning-fruits-vegetables.

37. "Toxins in Food," The Vulnerable Brain and Environmental Risks, vol. 2, edited by R. L. Isaacson and K. F. Jensen (New York: Plenum Press, 1992), np.

38. A. Adhikari, V. S. Chhetri, D. Bhattacharya, C. Cason, P. Luu, A. Suazo, "Effectiveness of daily rinsing of alfalfa sprouts with aqueous chlorine dioxide and ozonated water on the growth of Listeria monocytogenes during sprouting," PubMed, October 2019. See https://pubmed.ncbi.nlm.nih.gov/31429475/. Alfalfa sprouts have been implicated in multiple food-borne disease outbreaks. Significance and impact of the study: Sprouts are high-risk foods. Consumption of raw sprouts is frequently associated with food-borne disease outbreaks.

39. Circumcision: "And he that is eight days old shall be circumcised among you, every man child in your generations, he that is born in the house, or bought with money of any stranger, which is not of thy seed" (Genesis 17:12).

40. "Tongue and Lip Ties," La Leche League International's website. See https://www.llli.org/breastfeeding-info/tongue-lip-ties/.

41. Hoon Young Choi, M.D., Hyeong Cheon Park, M.D., and Sung Kyu Ha, M.D, "Salt Sensitivity and Hypertension: A Paradigm Shift from Kidney Malfunction to Vascular Endothelial Dysfunction," Electrolyte Blood Press, June 13, 2015, 7–16.

42. Jenna Fletcher, "Everything You Need to Know about Infant Botulism," Medical News Today, July 1, 2019. See https://www.medicalnewstoday.com/articles/325626.

43. See https://www.cdc.gov/botulism/index.html. Accessed December 14, 2020.

44. See https://health.gov/our-work/food-nutrition for up-to-date dietary guidelines. Accessed December 14, 2020.

45. According to the American Academy of Pediatrics (a subscription website), 77 children each year choke to death in an effort to eat hot dogs. See https://safekids.org/safetytips/field_risks/choking-and-strangulation. Accessed December 15, 2020.

46. N.E. Emmerik, F. de Jong, R. M. Elburg, "Dietary Intake of Sodium during Infancy and the Cardiovascular Consequences Later in Life: A Scoping Review," Karger, 2020. See https://www.karger.com/Article/FullText/507354.

47. Henry F. Hoffman, DDS, "Results of Premature Loss of Deciduous Teeth," International Journal of Orthodontia, Volume 1, Issue 2, February 1915, pages 47–57, American Association of Orthodontists. See https://www.sciencedirect.com/science/article/abs/pii/S1072347115800364?via%3Dihub. Accessed December 14, 2020.

48. See "Vitamin C for the Common Cold," WebMD Medical Reference, reviewed by Jennifer Robinson, MD, on May 13, 2019, WebMD; https://www.webmd.com/cold-and-flu/cold-guide/vitamin-c-for-common-cold#2.

49. N. Khandpur, J. Charles, R. E. Blaine, C. Blake, and K. Davison, "Diversity in fathers' food parenting practices: A qualitative exploration within a heterogeneous sample," Appetite, June 1, 2016, 134–45.

50. Natalie D. Muth, "Recommended Drinks for Young Children Ages 0–5," HealthyChildren.org, Sept. 18, 2019. See https://www.healthychildren.org/English/healthy-living/nutrition/Pages/Recommended-Drinks-for-Young-Children-Ages-0-5.aspx.

51. Richard Klasco, M.D., "Is There Such a Thing as a 'Sugar High'?" New York Times, February 25, 2020. Many parents blame sugar for their children's

hyperactive behavior. But the myth has been debunked. See https://www.nytimes.com/2020/02/21/well/eat/is-there-such-a-thing-as-a-sugar-high.html#:~:text=Many%20parents%20blame%20sugar%20for,the%20myth%20has%20been%20debunked. Accessed December 15, 2020.

52. Victor W. Zhong, Linda Van Horn, and Marilyn C. Cornelius et al., "Associations of Dietary Cholesterol or Egg Consumption With Incident Cardiovascular Disease and Mortality," PubMed.gov, March 19, 2019. See https://pubmed.ncbi.nlm.nih.gov/30874756/.

53. Nihon Ishigaku Zasshi, "Dutch Research on Beriberi: I. Christiaan Eijkman's Research and Evaluation of Kanehiro Takaki's Diet Reforms of the Japanese Navy," PubMed, March 2017. See https://pubmed.ncbi.nlm.nih.gov/30549780/. Accessed December 15, 2020.

54. "Eating white rice regularly may raise the 2 diabetes risk," Harvard School of Public Health. The study was first published in the *British Medical Journal* March 15, 2012. See https://www.hsph.harvard.edu/news/hsph-in-the-news/eating-white-rice-regularly-may-raise-type-2-diabetes-risk/.

55. Alireza Ostadrahimi et al., "Aflatoxin in Raw and Salt-Roasted Nuts (Pistachios, Peanuts, and Walnuts)," NCBI, January 7, 2014. See https://www.ncbi.nlm.nih.gov/pmc/articles/PMC4138677/. Accessed December 15, 2020.

56. See Wikipedia, https://en.wikipedia.org/wiki/Lipid_hypothesis, for more information on the Lipid Hypothesis.

57. "32% of pupils skip breakfast before school, study finds," *The Guardian*, August 15, 2010. See https://www.theguardian.com/society/2010/aug/16/third-pupils-skip-breakfast.

58. For the World Health Organization's Vitamin and Mineral Requirements, visit https://apps.who.int/iris/bitstream/handle/10665/42716/9241546123.pdf and download their booklet.

59. Margaret C Duellman, Judith M Lukaszuk, Aimee D Prawitz, and Jason P Brandenburg, "Protein supplement users among high school athletes have misconceptions about effectiveness," PubMed.gov, July 22, 2008. See https://pubmed.ncbi.nlm.nih.gov/18545198/. Accessed December 15, 2020.

60. In an overview of DHEA, the Mayo Clinic reported that it might reduce high-density lipoprotein (HDL), or "good," cholesterol levels. Use of DHEA also might worsen psychiatric disorders and increase the risk of mania in people who have mood disorders. DHEA also might cause oily skin, acne, and unwanted, male-pattern hair growth in women (hirsutism). See https://www.mayoclinic.org/drugs-supplements-dhea/art-20364199.

61. Lin Ding et al., "Trimethylamine-N-oxide (TMAO)-induced atherosclerosis is associated with bile acid metabolism," PubMed.gov., December 19, 2018. See https://pubmed.ncbi.nlm.nih.gov/30567573/. Accessed December 15, 2020.

62. Deborah Weatherspoon, "What should my cholesterol level be at my age?," Medical News Today, January 5, 2020. See https://www.medicalnewstoday.com/articles/315900.

63. In spite of many claims found in best-selling nutrition books, no scientific cause and effect relationship has been established between diet and breast cancer.

64. David Hurst, "Healthy eating can make tummy trouble WORSE: Why a high-fibre diet isn't always the answer for gut problems," Journal of the American Dietetic Association, June 2010. See https://www.dailymail.co.uk/health/article-2249651/Healthy-eating-make-tummy-trouble-WORSE-Why-high-fibre-diet-isnt-answer-gut-problems.html.

65. "Vitamin B: Fact Sheet for Consumers," National Institutes of Health, December 10, 2019. Recent research has demonstrated that, while water-soluble vitamins from food cannot generally reach dangerous levels, supplements should still be used with caution. The latest recommendations from the National Academy of Sciences (NAS), for example, call for 1.3 to 1.7 milligrams of vitamin B-6. Although some people claim a very high intake of vitamin B-6 can produce valuable health benefits, doses greater than 100 milligrams have caused nerve damage and are listed as a health risk in the new NAS recommendations. The report also warns of toxic effects from excessive doses of niacin. See https://ods.od.nih.gov/factsheets/VitaminB6-Consumer/. Accessed December 16, 2020.

66. These members of the B complex are not considered to be vitamins in humans.

67. "New Research Sheds Light on How UV Rays May Contribute to Cataracts," National Eye Institute, June 3, 2014. See https://www.nei.nih.gov/about/news-and-events/news/new-research-sheds-light-how-uv-rays-may-contribute-cataract.

68. Alan K. Silverman et al.,"Hypervitaminosis A syndrome: A paradigm of retinoid side effects," Journal of the American Academy of Dermatology, Volume 16, Issue 5, Part 1, May 1987, pages 1027–1039. See Science Direct, https://www.sciencedirect.com/science/article/abs/pii/S0190962287701339.

69. Dipen Khoosal and Ran D. Goldman, "Vitamin E for treating children's scars: Does it help reduce scarring?," Canada Family Physician, July 10, 2006, 52(7): 855–56.

70. "Dietary Supplements Fail to Prevent Prostate Cancer," December 15, 2008; NIH Research study. See https://www.nih.gov/news-events/nih-research-matters/dietary-supplements-fail-prevent-prostate-cancer. Accessed December 14, 2020.

71. Agnese Gugliandolo, Placido Bramanti, and Emanuela Mazzon, "Role of Vitamin E in the Treatment of Alzheimer's Disease," Nov 23, 2017. See https://www.ncbi.nlm.nih.gov/pmc/articles/PMC5751107/#:~:text=A%20

systematic%20review%20concluded%20that,effects%20or%20mortality%20%5B81%5D. Accessed December 14, 2020.

72. E. Herold, J. Mottin, Z. Savry, "Effect of vitamin E on human sexual functioning," PubMed, Sept. 8, 1979. See https://pubmed.ncbi.nlm.nih.gov/496621/.

73. Gunda Siska, Vitamin D Helps the Immune System During Cold and Flu Season," Pharmacy Times, Sept. 20, 2020. See https://www.pharmacytimes.com/news/vitamin-d-helps-the-immune-system-during-cold-and-flu-season.

74. Asma M. Alakiabi and Naser A. Alsharairi, "Current Evidence on Vitamin D Deficiency and Metabolic Syndrome in Obese Children: What Does the Evidence from Saudi Arabia Tell Us?" mdpi.com, Nov. 11, 2017. See https://www.mdpi.com/2227-9067/5/1/11.

75. "A common mutation in the MTHFR gene is a risk factor for non syndromic cleft lip and palate anomalies," *Iranian Journal of Otorhinolaryngology,* Jan. 27, 2015. See https://www.ncbi.nlm.nih.gov/pmc/articles/PMC4344969/#:~:text=The%20presence%20of%20the%20C677T,and%20non%2Dsyndromic%20cleft%20palates. Accessed December 14, 2020.

76. From the author's previously published work with M.Tolaroval.

77. "Magnesium Supplements May Help Lower High Blood Pressure," American Heart Association, August 20, 1998. Researchers at the National Cardiovascular Center in Osaka, Japan, found that daily magnesium supplements of 480 mg decreased blood pressure in Japanese adults with high blood pressure. See Science Daily, https://www.sciencedaily.com/releases/1998/08/980824071607.htm.

78. From the author's clinical work with Neo-Mull-Soy.

79. Ibid.

80. Trihalomethanes (THM) are a family of chemicals formed during the chlorination process used in most municipal water systems nationwide. Trihalomethanes form when chlorine reacts with organic matter or with components of sea water. The EPA has been considering a stricter standard for trihalomethanes because exposure to the contaminant has also been linked to an increased risk of cancer. The study was led by Waller and Shanna Swann, an epidemiologist with the state Department of Health Services. The EPA helped fund the study.

81. Richard J. Summerhayes et al., "Exposure to trihalomethanes in drinking water and small-for-gestational-age births," PubMed, Jan. 2012. See https://pubmed.ncbi.nlm.nih.gov/22157301/.

82. Melissa Denchak, "Flint Water Crisis: Everything You Need to Know," NRDC, Nov. 8, 2018. See https://www.nrdc.org/stories/flint-water-crisis-everything-you-need-know.

83. Jáuregui-Lobera, "Iron deficiency and cognitive functions," NCBI, Nov. 10, 2014. Baumgartner et al. found that in children with poor iron and n-3 fatty

acid status, iron supplementation improved verbal and nonverbal learning and memory, particularly in children with anemia. See https://www.ncbi.nlm. nih.gov/pmc/articles/PMC4235202/. Accessed December 14, 2020.

84. Harri Hemilä, "Zinc lozenges and the common cold: a meta-analysis comparing zinc acetate and zinc gluconate, and the role of zinc dosage," PubMed, May 8, 2017. See https://pubmed.ncbi.nlm.nih.gov/28515951/. Accessed December 14, 2020.

85. Patrick J. Skerrett, *Harvard Health*, "Zinc for the common cold? Not for me." See https://www.health.harvard.edu/blog/zinc-for-the-common-cold-not-for-me-201102171498, posted February 17, 2011 and updated March 6, 2020. Accessed December 14, 2020.

86. Melissa Jenco, "AAP continues to recommend fluoride following new study on maternal intake and child IQ," *AAP News*, August 19, 2019. See https://www.aappublications.org/news/2019/08/19/fluoride081919. Accessed December 14, 2020.

87. Daniel Pendick, "New study links L-carnitine in red meat to heart disease," Harvard Health, April 17, 2013. See https://www.health.harvard.edu/blog/new-study-links-l-carnitine-in-red-meat-to-heart-disease-201304176083. Accessed December 16, 2020.

88. "The New Nutrition Facts Label: What's in It for You?," U.S. Food and Drug Administration, June 29, 2020. See https://www.fda.gov/food/nutrition-education-resources-materials/new-nutrition-facts-label. Accessed December 16, 2020.

89. Anna Hinds, "How to Store and Cook Leftover Vegetables," September 24, 2020. See http://www.storingandfreezing.co.uk/how-store-cook-leftover-vegetables.html. Accessed December 14, 2020.

Index

About the Author

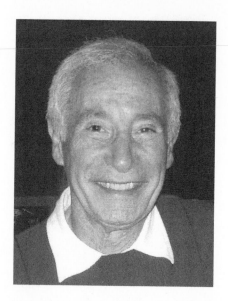

Dr. Goldberg was the founder of San Rafael Pediatrics in San Rafael, California. He was affiliated with Marin General Hospital in Marin County, California and California Pacific Medical Center in San Francisco.

In 2001 Doctor Goldberg was selected as one of fifty "Unsung Heroes Of Compassion" from around the world and was acknowledged personally by His Holiness the XIV Dalai Lama